"*Play Therapy and Expressive Arts in a Complex and Dynamic World: Opportunities and Challenges Inside and Outside the Playroom*" co-edited by Isabella Cassina, Claudio Mochi, and Karen Stagnitti is an innovative and much-needed book. It takes us into the realm of today's complex world addressing crisis situations, Covid, tele-health and the need for being in nature. Readers are treated to the expertise of internationally renowned authors who offer in-depth practical and useful guidance for working with children and adults. This is a much-needed addition to the professional library of beginner and experienced clinicians alike.

Athena A. Drewes, *PsyD, RPT-S*
Licensed Psychologist and Registered Play Therapist Supervisor
Founder and President Emeritus of the New York
Association for Play Therapy
Past Director of the Association for Play Therapy
Ocala, Florida, US

This exciting book by a distinguished group of contributors takes play therapy outside of its comfort zone to telehealth, crisis-disaster areas, high-risk countries, refugees and asylum seekers, while enlisting the healing power of nature. This excellent book is urgently needed!

David A. Crenshaw, *PhD, ABPP, RPT-S,*
author, Clinical Psychologist

Play Therapy and Expressive Arts in a Complex and Dynamic World

This book offers cutting-edge expertise and knowledge in new and developing play therapy, therapeutic play, and expressive arts for families and children in crisis and challenging situations.

The book focuses on the use of play therapies in complex and dynamic situations such as pandemics, post-disaster conditions, crisis, migration, poverty, and deprivation. Evidence in the book is rooted in theory and contains examples of direct clinical experiences of play therapy approaches by the authors from across six continents, offering innovative methods to apply expressive arts modalities across different situations. It highlights the need to understand the context and needs of the children and families in their particular situations and provides examples of application of therapeutic principles and techniques in individual and group settings and within schools and communities.

With reflections and guidance on how to support children in reaching their potential in a variety of difficult contexts, the book will be key reading for scholars and researchers in the fields of play therapy, expressive arts therapies, and creative psychotherapy, as well as professionals in these areas.

Isabella Cassina is Social Worker specialised in International Cooperation (IHEID Geneva) and Migration and Registered Therapeutic Play Specialist (APT Italy). She is International Speaker, Head of Project Management, and Trainer at the International Academy for Play Therapy (INA) in Switzerland.

Claudio Mochi is Clinical Psychologist, Child and Adolescents Psychotherapist, and Registered Play Therapist Supervisor.

Karen Stagnitti is Emeritus Professor at Deakin University, Australia, Occupational Therapist, and Play Therapist.

Routledge Research in Early Childhood Education

This series provides a platform for researchers to present their latest research and discuss key issues in Early Childhood Education.

Books in the series include:

Local Literacies in Early Childhood
Inequalities in place, policy and pedagogy
Helen Victoria Smith

Early Childhood Education in Germany
Exploring Historical Developments and Theoretical Issues
Edited by Bianca Bloch, Melanie Kuhn, Marc Schulz, Wilfried Smidt, and Ursula Stenger

Early Childhood Teachers' Professional Competence in Mathematics
Edited by Simone Dunekacke, Aljoscha Jegodtka, Thomas Koinzer, Katja Eilerts and Lars Jenßen

Decisions and Dilemmas of Research Methods in Early Childhood Education
Edited by Anne Keary, Janet Scull, Susanne Garvis and Lucas Walsh

Play Therapy and Expressive Arts in a Complex and Dynamic World
Opportunities and Challenges Inside and Outside the Playroom
Edited by Isabella Cassina, Claudio Mochi, and Karen Stagnitti

For more information about this series, please visit: www.routledge.com/education/series/RRECE

Play Therapy and Expressive Arts in a Complex and Dynamic World

Opportunities and Challenges Inside and Outside the Playroom

Edited by Isabella Cassina,
Claudio Mochi, and
Karen Stagnitti

Routledge
Taylor & Francis Group

LONDON AND NEW YORK

First published 2023
by Routledge
4 Park Square, Milton Park, Abingdon, Oxon OX14 4RN

and by Routledge
605 Third Avenue, New York, NY 10158

Routledge is an imprint of the Taylor & Francis Group, an informa business

British Library Cataloguing-in-Publication Data
A catalogue record for this book is available from the British Library

Library of Congress Cataloging-in-Publication Data
Names: Cassina, Isabella, 1984– editor. | Mochi, Claudio, editor. |
    Stagnitti, Karen, editor.
Title: Play therapy and expressive arts in a complex and dynamic world :
    opportunities and challenges inside and outside the playroom / edited by
    Isabella Cassina, Claudio Mochi, Karen Stagnitti.
Description: Milton Park, Abingdon, Oxon ; New York, NY : Routledge,
    2023. | Series: Routledge research in early childhood education |
    Includes bibliographical references and index.
Identifiers: LCCN 2022009405 (print) | LCCN 2022009406 (ebook) |
    ISBN 9781032169378 (hardback) | ISBN 9781032172323 (paperback) |
    ISBN 9781003252375 (ebook)
Subjects: LCSH: Play therapy.
Classification: LCC RJ505.P6 P5282 2023 (print) | LCC RJ505.P6 (ebook) |
    DDC 618.92/891653—dc23/eng/20220528
LC record available at https://lccn.loc.gov/2022009405
LC ebook record available at https://lccn.loc.gov/2022009406

ISBN: 978-1-032-16937-8 (hbk)
ISBN: 978-1-032-17232-3 (pbk)
ISBN: 978-1-003-25237-5 (ebk)

DOI: 10.4324/9781003252375

Typeset in Bembo
by Apex CoVantage, LLC

Contents

List of contributors   ix

Introduction   1
ISABELLA CASSINA

1   **Applying the therapeutic power of play and
    expressive arts in contemporary crisis work:
    a process-oriented approach**   6
    ISABELLA CASSINA AND CLAUDIO MOCHI

2   **Integrating creative arts modalities in the playroom
    and outside: live and remote interventions**   28
    STEVE HARVEY

3   **Recovering lost play time: principles and intervention
    modalities to address the psychosocial wellbeing of
    asylum seekers and refugee children**   50
    ISABELLA CASSINA

4   **Tele-Play Therapy: principles of remote interventions
    using the therapeutic powers of play**   69
    KATE L. RENSHAW AND JUDI A. PARSON

5   **Learn to Play Therapy in high-risk countries:
    the example of Nigeria**   96
    CLAUDIO MOCHI AND KAREN STAGNITTI

6   **Nature-based Play Therapy interventions in the digital age**   120
    MAGGIE FEARN

7 **Play and expressive arts to enhance professional development and personal growth in challenging contexts** 138

CLAUDIO MOCHI, STEVE HARVEY, AND ISABELLA CASSINA

Index 159

Contributors

Isabella Cassina, MA, TP-S, CAGS (Expressive Arts Therapy), PhD Candidate, is Social Worker specialised in International Cooperation (IHEID Geneva) and Migration and Registered Therapeutic Play Specialist (Association for Play Therapy Italy (APTI)). She is International Speaker, Head of Project Management, and Trainer at the International Academy for Play Therapy (INA) in Switzerland.

Maggie Fearn, MA DATP, MA HIPPT, is Humanistic and Integrative Child Psychotherapist, British Association of Play Therapists (BAPT) Play Therapist and Clinical Supervisor, Senior Lecturer, University of South Wales and the Children's Therapy Centre, Eire. She is affiliated with Senior Fellow Higher Education Academy. Her clinical practice with children and their families is developmental and trauma informed. Her research explores the evidence base for Nature-based Play Therapy interventions.

Steve Harvey, PhD, RPT-S, BC-DMT, RDT, is currently consulting in schools and is an adjunct faculty member in the Clinical Psychology Department at the University of Guam. He has been an active contributor to the integration of expressive modalities in Play Therapy. He helped pioneer the field of Family Play Therapy.

Claudio Mochi, MA, RP, RPT-S, is Psychotherapist, Director of the training program at the INA in Switzerland, and Founder of the APTI. He has conducted trainings and projects in the disaster mental health field internationally and presented on Play Therapy and trauma in six continents and over 20 countries.

Judi A. Parson, PhD, MA Play Therapy, is Paediatric Qualified Registered Nurse, Play Therapist/Supervisor, Discipline Lead, and Senior Lecturer in Play Therapy. She is affiliated with Deakin University. As an academic, she has authored/edited over 30 publications, continues to provide clinical and research supervision, and offers Play Therapy services, face-to-face and online.

Kate L. Renshaw, B. Psych, Grad. Cert. HELT, Grad. Dip. Art Therapy, Grad. Dip. Play Therapy, PhD Candidate, is Play and Filial Therapist, Supervisor, and Academic at Deakin University. She holds registrations with BAPT (RPT), APPTA (RPT/S), and APT (International Professional). Kate works therapeutically with children, families, and teachers.

Karen Stagnitti, PhD, BOccThy, GCHE, is Emeritus Professor in the School of Health and Social Development at Deakin University, Geelong, Australia. She has over 40 years of experience in clinical practice with children and families and research and teaching at the university level. She has over 140 publications.

Introduction

Isabella Cassina

The world is complex and dynamic with few certainties and a great number of emerging needs and conditions. Professionals from mental health and psychoeducational fields working with children, adolescents, and families are required to constantly expand their knowledge and nurture personal awareness. This book aims to provide students and professionals with insights and practical tools for daily use. A careful selection of Play Therapy methodologies, play-based and expressive arts activities, psychosocial projects, and clinical case studies is presented to stimulate readers' constructive reflection on their role as an agent of change, understanding their clients' needs, and planning for their own interventions.

The chapters are written on the basis of the clinical and non-clinical experience of professionals specialised in play therapy and expressive/creative arts therapy. Play therapy is "the systematic use of a theoretical model to establish an interpersonal process wherein trained Play Therapists use the therapeutic powers of play to help clients prevent or resolve psychosocial difficulties and achieve optimal growth and development" (Association for Play Therapy, 2022). Drewes and Schaefer (2014: 2) defined the therapeutic powers of play as "the specific change agents in which play initiates, facilitates, or strengthens their therapeutic effect". "Therapeutic factors are the actual mechanism that effect change in clients" (Yalom, 1995; cited in Drewes and Schaefer, 2014: 1). Expressive Arts Therapy is "the purposeful use of movement, music, image-making, performance, writing, and play and imagination in healthcare, psychotherapy, and wellness" (Malchiodi, 2020).

Throughout the pages of this book, the reader is presented with the transformative and healing power of play and expressive arts in action in various cultural contexts and settings, inside and outside the playroom, live and remote. The experiences described are drawn from the work in six continents with the following common threads: (a) the focus on the process rather than specific techniques; (b) the attention on the conditions, needs, and assets of children and their families more than just their pathology or disorder; (c) the application of therapeutic principles and techniques both in "typical" individual and group settings and in larger settings such as schools and communities. The multitude of contexts explored expresses the flexibility of the application of play and

DOI: 10.4324/9781003252375-1

expressive arts and is intended to allow the reader to identify with the situations presented and/or to prepare for future experiences in the field.

Chapter 1[1] focuses on the application of the therapeutic power of play and expressive arts in contemporary crisis work. The chapter also has the function of enabling the reader to better understand the chapters that follow. The authors present the concept of "crisis" from a psychological and humanitarian perspective. Key elements are introduced to support the application of a process-oriented approach and the need for a co-created intervention with the aim of supporting people to be authors in shaping their lives and future. The elements described include the conception of crisis as the intersection between its nature, the characteristics of the individual and the support system, the shift from a *continuum* to *contiguum* logic, and the innovative concept of MAP (My Awareness Process).

After considerations on how to prepare for field work, the authors share the example of the process-oriented approach "Coping with the present while building for the future" (CPBF) supported by the Theatre Metaphor and a visual chart in which the elements (or actions) of an intervention or project are organised in chronological order. The concept of good practice (versus best practice) is presented as well as the grounding phase in crisis work, the key role of capacity building as a way to expand capabilities, opportunities, and choices, and the ideal time to apply the therapeutic powers of play, play therapy, and expressive arts. The actions described are enriched with practical examples from the field.

Chapter 2 presents an overview of how the practice of play therapy can be expanded to include creative art therapy (CAT) modalities as integrated actions within a cohesive intervention with children, their families, and in crisis situations. Typically, play therapy activity is presented as primarily conducted with children and involves a certain range of expressive activities such as play with toys, sand trays, or puppets. However, play activity can be extended to include adults, families, and the use of other expressive avenues such as drama, music, art, storytelling, and dance/movement interaction within the in-person playroom and online.

The use of several creative art modalities can facilitate therapeutic powers that are part of the natural experience of interactive play that contributes to the individual's development of an alliance, creativity, and an expansion of emotional expression. Mechanisms of change related to the CAT such as active involvement with symbolism, metaphor making, and the enjoyment that accompanies arts-based expression are reviewed. The chapter also addresses how this creative arts/play approach has been applied online with international adult participants in response to the Covid-19 health crisis as well as with families, especially in situations when a verbal understanding is complex.

Chapter 3 explores how to respond to the impact of forced displacement on children's psychosocial wellbeing. The phenomenon of migration is presented as a process where children face an accumulating number of difficulties that do not end once they reach the country where their families seek asylum. The author suggests the concept of "Recovering lost play time" as both the heart of the issue for children and the response that child professionals can apply in a variety of highly vulnerable situations.

The chapter is written from the perspective of a professional providing psychosocial support to children showing aggressiveness, lack of self-control and social competences, depression, anxiety, low self-esteem, hyperactivity, and developmental issues. The questions addressed in this chapter are: what do displaced children need most once they reach our service? How do we involve their families in the process? Why, when, and how do we introduce and use the therapeutic power of play and, more specifically, play therapy interventions? The answers to these questions unfold throughout the chapter by providing a theoretical orientation on children's psychosocial needs, a concrete example of a project developed in a reception centre by the author and her team, and a case study with a child in child-centred play therapy.

Chapter 4 is dedicated to an overview of the practice of Tele-Play Therapy. The authors underline that play therapy offered through the virtual environment is not a substitute for face-to-face therapy, but requires serious consideration of how virtual paediatric mental health service provision can be made safe, accessible, and a desirable option. The child and their family are the central focus to determine the level of Tele-Play Therapy intervention with seamless connectivity between the human and digital ecosystems.

In Section 1, the principles for remote Tele-Play Therapy are established. First, play therapists should initially familiarise themselves with the scaffolded approach to telecommunications for play therapy. The second step is reviewing the guiding principles that set out both practice guidelines and contraindications for using telecommunications in play therapy. The third is to consider and prepare the three Tele-Play Therapy practice environments, namely: the practitioner, the child client, and the virtual setting. Finally, a diverse range of telecommunications practice considerations is given. To highlight these principles in action, a composite case example is offered in Section 2. Henry is the focal point of this remote Tele-Play Therapy intervention; the therapeutic powers of play are aligned with his biopsychosocial health needs within the context of his family.

Chapter 5 provides an overview of Learn to Play Therapy and explores the application of this model in high-risk countries with both clinical and non-clinical populations. After introducing the general psychosocial conditions and challenges for youth and their families, the chapter provides a specific and practical example of a project developed in schools and daycare settings in Nigeria. The project aimed to strengthen the local support system as a means of widening the range of protective factors for children and their families.

The authors describe the key role of teachers and other local professionals in applying play and play therapy to create an optimal learning environment; foster fundamental skills in children such as narrative language ability, self-regulation, and emotional-social competence; and support children in reaching their potential and overcoming psychosocial problems. The gradual progression from introductory activities to more specialised activities is also presented highlighting the importance of adapting daily practice to identified needs. Case studies are provided to bring the content "alive" and illustrate the concrete application of the Learn to Play approach.

Chapter 6 considers the relevance and influence of the environment as the context for child development and therapeutic process in Nature-based Therapeutic Play and play therapy. The emergence in the infancy of embodied imagination through playful relationship and the developmental importance of being grounded in the body, in dynamic relationship with the environment, are explored.

The theoretical framework draws on the author's clinical practice and a synthesis of theory from human development, applied neurobiology, somatics, and psychodynamic theory and focuses on the role of nature as a therapeutic ally for the play therapist and child in the process of regulating and nourishing a child's sense of where they are, who they are, and what being safe feels like. The case study vignettes show that immersive play experiences in the natural environment promote a child's growth, development, and healing and evoke the possibilities, wonder, and limits of being a human being.

Chapter 7 offers an additional point of contact between all chapters of the book. It starts by sharing three main assumptions: a contemporary complex world requires professionals working with children, youths, and families, to have additional qualities and preparation to support client needs in circumstances of confusion, hostility, and sufferance; play and expressive arts have transformative and healing powers that can be expanded and respond effectively to new challenges; clear and safe boundaries can enhance professional development and nourish personal growth.

Section 1 introduces the *contiguum* of professional development-personal growth by presenting the basic components of a multi-phased approach in the framework applied to a project in India. This approach is supported by a diagram showing how the two processes of professional development and personal growth reinforce each other with the first giving progressively more space to the second. Section 2 focuses on creative collaborations between therapists in co-creating metaphors and overcoming shared challenges and discomfort. Two examples are provided: the first presents an online play space dedicated to professionals from around the world. The second is related to a supervision group in New Zealand who faced a difficult situation at work and decided to find new answers and meanings through an arts-based inquiry.

A book cannot contain all answers to current and future challenges, but it can be a *meeting point* for students and professionals from all over the world that encourages new responses and interventions. We hope that each chapter will stay with you long after you have closed the book, that the words you will read will turn into one or more actions allowing *you* to become even more aware of your value, and *your practice* to become even more effective.

Note

1 The descriptions of Chapters 1–7 have been elaborated by the authors of the chapters themselves.

References

Association for Play Therapy (2022) *Home page*, available: www.a4pt.org/ [accessed 26 January 2022].

Drewes, A.A. and Schaefer, C.E. (2014) 'Introduction. How play therapy causes therapeutic change', in C.E., Schaefer and A.A., Drewes (eds.) *The therapeutic powers of play: 20 core agents of change*, 2nd edn., Hoboken, NJ: Wiley, 1–7.

Malchiodi, C. (2020) *Expressive arts therapy and trauma: Using movement, sound, image, and performance to restore the self*, online conference for the United Nations in Geneva, Switzerland, June 2020, available: www.youtube.com/watch?v=SutB72QBvZs [accessed 6 December 2021].

1 Applying the therapeutic power of play and expressive arts in contemporary crisis work

A process-oriented approach

Isabella Cassina and Claudio Mochi

After considerations on how to prepare for field work, the authors share the example of the process-oriented approach "Coping with the present while building for the future" (CPBF) supported by the Theatre Metaphor and a visual chart in which the elements (or actions) of an intervention or project are organised in chronological order. The concept of good practice (versus best practice) is presented as well as the grounding phase in crisis work, the key role of capacity building as a way to expand capabilities, opportunities, and choices, and the ideal time to apply the therapeutic powers of play, play therapy, and expressive arts. The actions described are enriched with practical examples from the field.

Today, in this complex and dynamic world, the concept of "crisis" seems more actual than ever. This chapter starts by exploring this concept and providing a theoretical framework before diving into international field practice inside and outside the playroom.

The term "crisis" derives from Greek (κρίσις) and originally meant the "separation" (Ragaù, 2011). The term has agricultural beginnings (i.e. separating what was to keep from what was to eliminate during the grain harvest) and acquired secondary meanings as choose, judge, interpret, and decide. Over time, there has been a semantic shift towards a medically specific meaning with "crisis" described as the turning point in a disease, the moment in which the person with the disease could improve or worsen (Vocabulary.com, 2021).

In the field of Mental health, crisis has been described in different ways, with several elements in common. Crisis defines those events or circumstances that are perceived by the individual as intolerable (Gilliland and James cited in Mochi, 2009: 75–76) and stressful to the point of creating a sense of disruption to one's sense of balance. The situation is so overwhelming that usual coping abilities are not sufficient to re-establish a sense of safety and control and this creates functional impairments.

Certain situations represent a great "challenge for individuals' adaptive responses and coping capabilities" which can cause symptom formation and create a series of enduring personality changes (McFarlane and De Girolamo cited in VanFleet and Mochi, 2015). Nevertheless, "there is not an immediate and casual relationship between a specific event and individual reactions"

DOI: 10.4324/9781003252375-2

(op. cit.: 170). The same situation can produce crisis in one person and not in another.

Different authors (Caplan, 1964; Webb, 1999; Doherty, 2007; VanFleet and Mochi, 2015) point out that a crisis is the result of the interaction of different variables. Moreover, Webb (1999) maintains that each crisis should be assessed considering the nature of the circumstances, the idiosyncratic characteristics of each individual, and the strength and weakness of his support system (nuclear family, extended family, school, friends/community, culture/religion) (op. cit.: 5). According to Webb (op. cit.), "the impact of a specific situation depends on the balancing of the interacting influences among the three sets of variables".

Among the various conceptualisations and perspectives on crisis, Webb eloquently emphasises a crucial element for any intervention: the turning point for any individual is influenced not just by the characteristics of the situation but also by his/her perception of it, his/her capabilities, and the quality and effectiveness of the support he/she can receive. The most effective intervention is the one that helps and enhances the individual and their support system and, whenever possible, weakens the impact of the event. If ultimately "crisis is an individual response" and "exists IN the person" (Doherty, 2007: 3), it is also clear that there are external important factors to consider and work on.

The way crisis interventions are conceived depends on how the nature of the crisis itself is understood. In the past, for example, thinking of the crisis as a time-limited event or a "stress overload" situation (Webb, 2007: 6–7) was influential in structuring short-term interventions aimed at "returning to the previous state" (Doherty, 2007), "lessening the distress and anxiety and bolstering the coping skills" (Webb, 2007: 7). In many situations, this viewpoint still applies and early assistance helps to prevent the situation from getting worse (Caplan, 1964; Doherty, 2007; Webb, 2007). Alternative conceptualisations embrace a broader perspective that accommodates a wide variety of situations. In the next section, we will consider the humanitarian perspective on crisis.

THE HUMANITARIAN PERSPECTIVE ON CRISIS

In past decades, international humanitarian agencies have accumulated considerable experience in the world of crises that goes beyond the individual and have developed useful resources for professionals from different sectors. One reference tool is the Index for Risk Management (INFORM) developed through a collaboration between the Inter-Agency Standing Committee (IASC) Reference Group on Risk, Early Warning, and Preparedness and the European Commission. This Index guides professionals in understanding and monitoring the risk of humanitarian crises and disasters across all countries. This "can help identify where and why a crisis might occur, which means we can reduce the risk, build peoples' resilience and prepare better for when crises do happen" (IASC and EC, 2021a: 6).

The Index has three dimensions that synthesise information on risk. Each dimension has subcategories and a total of 80 different indicators. In order to compare countries, a risk profile is created for each country according to a rating where 0 is the absence of risk and 10 is the maximum level of risk.

The first dimension indicates the hazards and people's physical exposure to them and includes two subcategories: natural hazards and human-induced hazards. The second dimension is vulnerability of the predisposition of a population or community to be affected and destabilised by a hazard on economic, political, and social levels. Vulnerability includes two subcategories: socio-economic vulnerability of a country in general and vulnerable groups. The third dimension, also named "lack of coping capacity", is the availability of resources to sustain and develop people's coping capacity and, in general, increase the community's resilience. It includes institutional and infrastructure subcategories, where the first addresses mitigation and preparedness and the second addresses emergency response and recovery.

International agencies decide on the allocation of resources according to this Index. This tends to favour very high and high-risk countries; however, crises also happen in medium-risk countries (op. cit.: 20) and, as overwhelmingly demonstrated by the current pandemic, all countries have a potential for risk. That said, there is a big difference between countries (and regions in the same country) represented by the prerequisites, or "starting conditions", which are associated with two of the three dimensions: the level of vulnerability of the population and the availability of resources to sustain and develop people's coping capacity. In Chapters 3 and 5, crisis interventions are presented in Switzerland and Nigeria. Switzerland's risk class is "very low" (1,4) with a lack of coping capacities rated 0,9, which is extremely low. Nigeria's risk class is "very high" (6,5) with peaks in projected conflict risk (10), current highly violent conflict intensity (9), and a lack of coping capacity rated 6,5 (IASC and EC, 2021b).

Most of the time we cannot prevent natural and human disasters, but we can support people more effectively in overcoming the consequences of disasters and the whole community can be better prepared to face various and possible future critical events. This is where the psychological perspective meets the humanitarian perspective and lays the groundwork for our reasoning.

The variable of the "starting conditions" of a country is even more essential if we consider the change in crises in the last decades. Since the 1990s, the humanitarian world has had to rethink crises by abandoning the idea of a temporary transition (or a single critical episode that has a before and after) to embrace the reality that crises multiply, lengthen over time, and become more complex (Cassina, 2009). It is significant to know that "the average length of humanitarian crises has almost doubled over the past five years. An average humanitarian crisis now lasts for over nine years" (Joint Research Centre, 2020). One of the results of this recurrent phenomenon is the Forgotten crisis defined as "severe, protracted humanitarian crisis situations where affected populations are receiving no or insufficient international aid and where there is no political commitment to solve the crisis, due in part to a lack of media interest" (European Civil Protection and Humanitarian Aid Operations, 2021).

These kinds of crises are the result of difficult conditions and critical events that accumulate over time.

On a conceptual level, the world of international cooperation has made a transition from the logic of *continuum* to that of *contiguum*. This is a shift in thinking from a sequential and delimited conception and implementation of aid interventions (i.e. emergency-rehabilitation-development) to a recognition of all stages being complementary and simultaneous in time and space (Pirotte et al., 2000; Cassina, 2009). More recently, a third dimension called Nexus (which is the intersection of three sectors: humanitarian, development, and peacebuilding) was defined as "effectively addressing the needs and aspirations of people in protracted crises" (Carbonnier, 2019: 1). If we agree that "people affected by armed conflict obviously do not care whether the assistance they receive is labelled humanitarian or development" (United Nations General Assembly, 2017), then a synergy between emergency and development is needed.

Extraordinary events that happen to individuals are (or become) part of daily life for others (Mochi and Cassina, 2018). This does not mean that events don't impact people's lives and psychological wellbeing, but they could be perceived as "something normal that we can't do anything about". This reality underlines the need to consider crisis work as a co-creation with local partners throughout the process. After all, "both development and humanitarian organisations have long affirmed that participatory approaches involving 'beneficiaries' are key to ensuring the relevance and effectiveness of their interventions" (Carbonnier, 2019: 4–5).

This perspective brings us to a process-oriented approach or, even better, to the concept of MAP as suggested by Mochi (forthcoming 2022). MAP stands for "My Awareness Process" and outlines key principles to guide practitioners in designing an intervention according to their experience, certain criteria, and rules of action while maintaining maximum flexibility and space for co-construction. "A MAP is more like a collection of reference points, like the constellations for the sailors" that help to navigate uncharted waters. "It is not a precise plan to implement, nor a defined project one can use in every circumstance and country. It is neither a detailed travel book. No one can predict and dictate every single step that has to be taken" (op. cit.).

A process-oriented approach

We will now explain a practical approach to crisis intervention, focusing on the point of view of psychological wellbeing of children, families, and local professionals. First, we would like to share with the reader an activity, which we include in our trainings on this topic, to assist the reader to enter the perspective of international field work which, inevitably, raises deep emotions and reflections.

The activity is called "Arriving in Haiti". It involves a narrator, who reads and paces the story, so the group has time to understand and mime (possibly with broad and explicit movements) the story, step by step. The participants silently follow the story and enact what they hear in any way they wish, preferably while standing. This activity can be done both in-person and online and should ideally be followed by a discussion in pairs or small groups about what was experienced. After this first reading, additional inputs and guidance from the presenters/trainers are given to trigger a process of co-construction of understanding of the context described.

Arriving in Haiti

I was assigned to a post-disaster psychosocial program, and I am currently in the aeroplane looking out of the window.

I am trying to glimpse the Caribbean sea but I am disappointed, I don't see anything but clouds.

I have been on this aeroplane for 10 hours and my backside hurts very much.

This is the third flight, and my shirt doesn't smell so fresh.

Oh, we are finally landing! I am so excited.

Getting off the aeroplane, I feel so hot. It is like having a giant dryer right in front of my face.

I look around trying to see where the shuttle bus is when suddenly. . . . I am packed inside a mini vehicle with many other sweaty people.

After waiting for a long time in a sort of garage, I receive my suitcase back. I am glad.

Leaving the airport I have at least 30 people around me; they all want to assist me by grabbing my luggage; I feel hands everywhere.

I run out from the crowd, and finally, I reach the outside of the gate where I take a deep breath.

I can read my name on a piece of paper, somebody is waiting for me, and I feel relieved.

I am now in the car, and I see rubble everywhere; there is not even a building that is not destroyed.

Naked children are moving quickly through the garbage. People of all ages are walking in the middle of the street, we have to be very careful and slow down.

My shirt is incredibly sticky, my eyes are burning, and I have never felt so thirsty.

We keep on driving; I see nothing but rubble everywhere and thousands of tents and thousands of people. There is desperation everywhere.

I feel overwhelmed. I am trying to focus my mind on what we will do first thing tomorrow. What can we do for all these people?

Finally, we arrive at the camp. There is dust and the smell of plastic on fire, it is so hot here, and my bags are heavy.

I am exhausted, but I will spend the rest of the day in briefings while I keep thinking: "Where will we start tomorrow?"

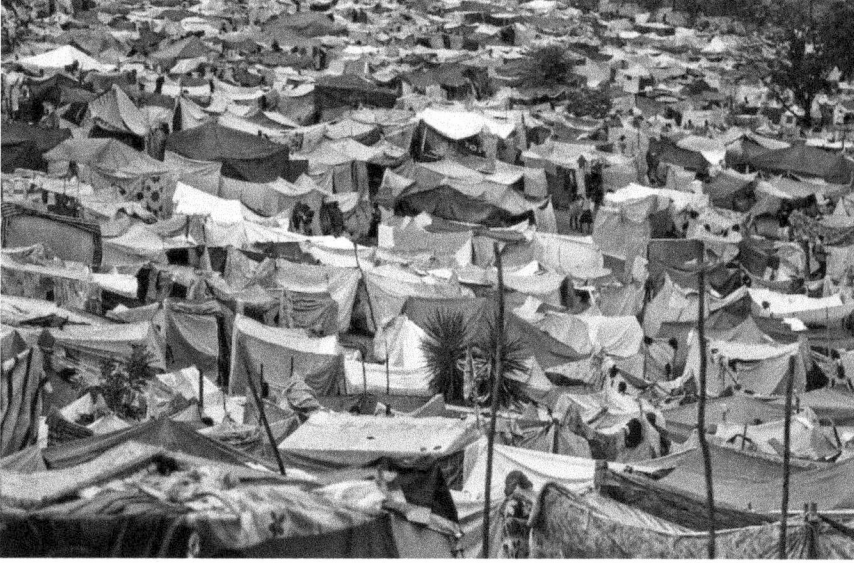

Figure 1.1 A glimpse of Port-au-Prince, Haiti's capital, after the earthquake in 2010.
Source: Photograph by Claudio Mochi.

The starting point: preparing for field work

The preparation of crisis field professionals starts before the trigger event happens or their arrival in a foreign country. The preparation includes both personal and professional dimensions. The personal dimension is a complete (or at least advanced ongoing) process of self-knowledge and self-awareness, strengthening a number of fundamental skills including empathic listening, self-control, and flexibility with particular attention to creativity and playfulness (see Chapter 7).

The professional dimension is related to training and supervision in key areas such as programme and project cycle management, principles of international cooperation (if applicable), nature of the crisis and possible evolution, resources and limits of the support system in the country or region, specific cultural perspectives and issues, particularities related to the area of intervention (psychological, social, educational, health, or rehabilitation), and approaches, methodologies, and techniques in specific fields. The authors of this chapter are trained in several methodologies applicable to crisis including trauma interventions. In their professional experience, supported by extensive literature, play therapy and expressive arts (both as therapy and as means to achieve and maintain wellbeing) proved to be particularly effective.

As well as the "before the crisis" preparation, additional considerations must be thought through carefully. First, crisis interventions can cause damage. "In the 1990s, several studies showed that humanitarians can inadvertently do harm while seeking to do good" (Anderson cited in Carbonnier, 2019: 4). The IASC lists "humanitarian aid-induced social problems" as one of the problem categories following a disaster (IASC, 2007). Crises are turning points in very complex, delicate, and painful situations, and different kinds of interventions can make situations better or worst. For instance, the participation of mental health professionals who do not belong to the community is discouraged, so the intervention can be "grounded locally" and "within a structure that can ensure the intervention duration and perspective" (VanFleet and Mochi, 2015: 175). Even though foreign professionals have previous experiences in crises, their contribution is advised to be focusing on supporting programmes on a general level and avoiding the direct implementation of interventions (IASC, 2007: 73–74).

Second, there are many orientations and approaches. The first task for each professional is to "separate" (κρίνω), to make a choice by selecting the most suitable intervention considering risks and benefits. We can imagine two extremes: (1) technical intervention and (2) process-oriented approaches. In the first case, the emphasis is on choosing the type of technique, approach, or protocol. It is a specialised form of intervention, based on the presumption that the most relevant and pressing needs are known and the most effective response is identified. The risk is, for instance, that stress management, trauma-focused interventions, fun, or entertainment is delivered without a real pre- or post-intervention. If we consider Figure 1.1, which single protocol could possibly meet all needs of the people going through such conditions unless it is part of a bigger plan? Crisis situations need high levels of care and effective and sustainable practices. At the same time, it is important to be aware that even the best practices risk the neglect of many necessities (IASC, 2007) and sometimes create profound resentments (VanFleet and Mochi, 2015). Moreover, especially in larger crises, a restricted number of individuals need specialised treatment and seldom access it in the first phases of the intervention (Brymer et al., 2006; IASC, 2007).

A process-oriented approach assumes that chaining of actions and different phases are necessary to understand the variety of needs and resources available, adaptation to the evolving aspects of the context, and engagement and cooperation with the local support system. We provide an example of the process-oriented approach in this chapter. If you, the reader, have the impression that crisis work is quite complicated, you are right. Let's summarise before proceeding:

- Crises are increasingly complex, severe, and protracted. They result from the intersection of three main components: nature of the crisis, individual factors (or people's vulnerability), and conditions of the support system (or level of community's coping capacity).
- The individuals and their context cannot be separated and this is why working on the support system is pivotal.
- Every country (or region) can be potentially in crisis, but the "starting conditions" make the difference in how we face and overcome it (resources

available, timing, etc.). In any case, the crisis intervention must be co-created with local partners.

- The general aim of crisis work is to improve people's life conditions and improve future perspectives. Sometimes restoring the "previous" conditions is neither feasible nor optimal. That is why co-creation is even more important.
- Crisis professionals are required to have a combination of a high level of self-awareness, preparation, and flexibility. Critical contexts are unpredictable and potentially traumatic. Professionals must be ready to cope.

Coping with the present while building for the future

The approach "Coping with the present while building for the future" (or "CPBF") (Mochi and Cassina, 2018) is the result of a theoretical synthesis that draws its origin from international field practice, which developed in collaboration with a multitude of local actors. This approach must be seen as a MAP in the terms suggested by Mochi (forthcoming 2022). In fact, crises scenarios are different and unique. If pre-packed interventions can be dangerous, so too can having no references at all.

A MAP is the awareness of process and knowledge that each professional or organisation should bring with them as they move into unknown critical scenarios. A MAP assists to sustain partners and local professionals in gaining a sense of safety, orientation, and understanding in confusing or dangerous times. A MAP includes all necessary elements that support the co-construction of the entire crisis intervention. Figure 1.2 presents the points that constitute the authors' process of awareness. We are going to explore the elements that give a clearer picture of the nature of the intervention and may facilitate the comprehension of the concepts expressed throughout this book.

> Imagine the crisis intervention as a co-construction of a stage upon which to narrate and produce different plays. . . . The first act is a source of inspiration for the second. . . . Every day you play and pick up all sensitive information while building the base for the next act. In this way the play is always responsive and engaging. The intervention is a co-created developing story that cannot be rushed.
>
> (Mochi, forthcoming 2022)

The Theatre Metaphor (Mochi and Cassina, 2018) underlines the nature of the intervention, which should be organised and creative at the same time. Crisis professionals must not act out their own script. Rather, they use their expertise and flexibility to facilitate the co-creation and the progression of all necessary operations that leads to "support individuals and communities to have their own theatre" where they can "uncover their past stories and decide which future plays they want to perform" and then to support their acting (op. cit.).

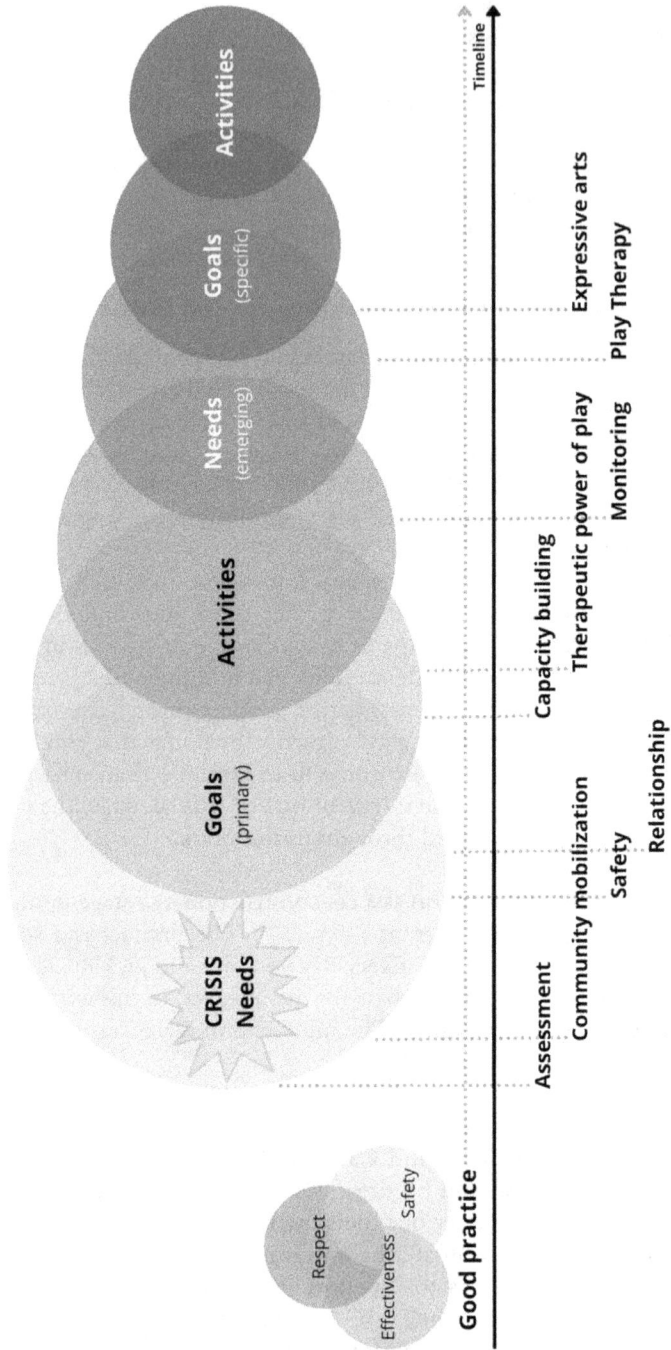

Figure 1.2 The approach "Coping with the present while building for the future" (CPBF).

A guide to understanding and reading the CPBF chart

Figure 1.2 (referred to as "CPBF chart") illustrates the structure of the crisis intervention by organising the elements of the authors' MAP in a chronological order, which then translates into an order of action. Within the framework of a process, some elements are placed before others on the timeline and, therefore, must be implemented earlier.

The lower part of the CPBF chart

The initial assessment is dedicated to gathering information about the purpose of the intervention, and the immediate concerns and needs focusing on the primary and most pressing necessities (Brymer et al., 2006). During this phase, professionals can also pursue other objectives such as establishing human connections, enhancing immediate and ongoing safety, providing physical and emotional comfort, and offering practical assistance. In this way, first contacts can also function as a way to lay the foundation for positive relationships with local people, arouse interest in participating actively in initiatives, and provide ideas on possible solutions to the problems presented.

It is very difficult to engage somebody without having first established a connection and created a positive relationship, so the person feels safe with us. Elements on the timeline indicate an action (or a series of actions) that can be reached only if the preliminary actions have taken place. The placement on the timeline does not indicate the amount of time required before you can move on, and this time factor can vary a lot according to the nature of the crisis and the "starting conditions" of the country or region. For instance, reaching the moment for capacity building can take much more time in one context compared to another. In our project in Switzerland (see Chapter 3), capacity building for professionals in the migration field started as soon as the project was officially accepted. In Haiti, it took us months before starting capacity building because the disaster was devastating, and the support system was particularly fragile. Specific timings from one element to another are difficult to predict, in contrast to the chronological order of actions, which are clear and none can be skipped.

One more consideration is that the elements (or actions) must not be seen as something we do once and for all but something to maintain "from that moment on". We don't just do one needs assessment, we don't reach a feeling of safety and build a relationship once and for all, and we don't build capacities without giving a follow-up or adding further training if necessary.

The upper part of the CPBF chart

CPBF embraces a multilayered intervention framework where the progression of actions starts from the less specialised activities addressed to the larger population (represented by the bigger circles), to the most refined forms of treatment addressed to smaller parts of the population (smaller circles). In fact, in many critical circumstances, anything related to survival and primary needs comes before psychological welfare (VanFleet and Mochi, 2015: 169). For psychological welfare, psychotherapy or specialised treatments are most often a priority for a few individuals (Brymer et al., 2006; IASC, 2007).

Moreover, the CPBF chart underlines the continual logical order (or pattern) of "need-goal-activity" (or "N-G-A"). The crisis generates needs. In order to respond to these needs, it is necessary to establish common goals. In order to achieve these goals, we propose a series of activities. Since the assessment of needs is continuous (monitoring), it is likely that we will be able to detect emerging needs for which we will form new goals and propose new activities, and so on.

The good practice

Best practice comes after "good practice", which is the implementation of three elements in the field: respect, effectiveness, and safety (Mochi and Cassina, 2018). The term "respect" comes from the Latin verb *re-spicere*, which means literally "to look back". "Instead of proceeding forward" and going our own way, "we stop to give proper attention" (Mochi, forthcoming 2022). "Respect implies the need to take a moment to reflect, research, and evaluate doubts in order to apply what is considerate and courteous according to the situation" (op. cit.). Effectiveness is strictly related to respect. Reaching predefined goals is not enough. Good practice should enable the achievement of goals that are shared and "relevant" to people, and satisfy needs that are pertinent and carefully assessed.

In addition, in all possible scenarios, the priority should be "to stabilize the situation by helping individuals or groups to feel safe" (van der Kolk cited in Mochi, 2009: 77). Only "when the individual feels safe, he is ready to begin the course to regain psychic equilibrium and process his trauma, integrating traumatic memories, slowly recovering his self-regulation, re-establishing social connections, retrieving previously practised coping skills or learning new ones" (Mochi, 2009: 77).

In 1999, I (Claudio) was involved in my first crisis work. The direction I received was to use a specific protocol or a set of techniques. At the time, I did not realise that my supervisor had no more experience than I did. After several years, I have spent almost 3,000 days in the field with crises. When I feel disoriented I stop, look back and ask myself: "Am I respectful or have I jumped too fast into conclusions and unnecessary interventions? Am I really trying to understand and make space for others' perspective? Am I doing the most to support a sense of safety in people around me?"

Respect, effectiveness, and safety are interrelated and nourish each other on the common ground of relationship. It is through human connections that we can convey respect and support a sense of safety, and it is by showing respect and creating a feeling of safety that we build a stronger relationship. Through interactions with people who feel respected and safe, we are able to discover more about their needs and assets. What is important is to remember that good practice (such as the process of building a relationship) requires skill and time. This brings us back to the reasons for a process-oriented approach.

The grounding phase in crisis work

The MAP is a tool that provides orientation, promotes understanding, and supports professionals working in crisis. This tool is flexible and adaptable to many different contexts. It has been built on considerable field experience and follows a specific rationale. The elements of assessment, community mobilisation, safety, and relationship (grouped under the name "grounding phase") are preparatory for the advanced phase. Play therapy and expressive arts are extremely valuable in crisis situations, but in the CPBF approach, they are not included at the beginning. Paraphrasing a famous quote attributed to Plato, "we can discover more about a person in an hour of play than in a year of conversation". So why don't we use play right from the beginning? To answer this question, we will present two scenarios.

I (Claudio) have worked in a variety of contexts where, in the aftermath of a disaster, I was in contact with people who were extremely distressed and frightened. When I was in Lebanon in 2006, my assessment protocol included the possibility of organising a range of activities following the assessment. After becoming familiar with the parents, we created a temporary setting and expanded the evaluation of the children's psychological condition. I carried out my initial assessment in nine villages over 6 weeks.

Only one village had water and electricity. People were still missing and, even though not all families lost a member, almost everyone I interviewed had lost everything including their hope for a better future (Mochi, 2006). In the time I spent in the region, I rarely met children since they were kept safe at home, away from the fields filled with mines and falling buildings. I had meetings with hundreds of adults. All my energy and time were directed to collecting information on primary needs, determining the nature of the damage, and providing basic psychological support. I created connections with families and key people in the community, and I made my evaluation on the children's condition and needs, based on parents' and teachers' reports. During the weeks, because of the emotional climate, I never thought there was room for play activities.

In 2009, I (Isabella) was working in Belgrade, Serbia, in shelters for internally displaced persons (IDPs). The situation was characterised by poverty, mental illness, and intergenerational trauma. Over three decades, temporary shelters had become permanent residences and part of the population still relied on basic needs being supplied by local associations. In the area, the community was divided. I was in charge of the professional team who went to the field to gather information on needs and deliver basic necessities. At the same time, these visits were giving us pointers for developing longer-term projects in which to involve adults and families.

By the time I arrived in Serbia, local colleagues already had contacts with the community of IDPs and ideas on how to integrate them into the larger community. Nonetheless, the complexity of the situation was considerable. Humanitarian issues were intertwined with sociocultural, political, and economic ones. Before my first field visits, my colleagues instructed me to limit verbal interactions as my foreign accent could have been an additional source of scepticism and hostility. It took weeks before I was able to be fully emersed in field work. People were needy but alert, chronically stressed, and distrustful of local associations and even more of international collaborators. The children themselves, born and raised in the shelters, recounted endlessly how the war had destroyed their lives. The intergenerational trauma was evident.

Instead of implementing a pre-packaged plan of play and expressive arts activities, my focus was on understanding how I could be accepted by the community of IDPs and my own local colleagues. I was still far from the point where I could propose a collaboration with parents on children's play activities, parent–child activities, or adult-only activities. At that moment, it was impossible to show up in the field with toys and expressive materials. How to build the missing link?

Play and art are a universal language, but in a crisis context, we cannot "talk" with them from the beginning nor all the time. In the scenarios presented, we perceived that play, expressive arts, and other forms of specialised intervention were inappropriate to begin with and that some groundwork was necessary (isn't it the same worldwide when, for instance, we actively engage parents in the playroom?). Considerations on the topic are numerous, we put forward four main arguments:

1   *The hierarchy of needs must be respected.* Physiological and basic survival needs have priority as they are immediate of personal concern. It is tempting to assume that as mental health or humanitarian professionals, we know what is needed in critical circumstances (Mochi and VanFleet, 2009), but every situation and personal story is unique. Crises require understanding, not assuming. In complex situations, needs' assessment never ends and information is gathered across different circumstances (see Chapter 7 for an example of assessment in the field in India).

2   *Safety comes first.* If a person perceives the context as threatening or unsafe, his/her major preoccupation will be to protect him/herself. This can happen when he/she is completely overwhelmed, suspicious, does not know what to expect from the situation, or is simply new to certain experiences. We cannot make assumptions about people's sense of safety since our process to detect danger or threat works below our level of consciousness (Porges, 2011: 20). We can learn, explore, connect with others, play, create, and access our resources only when we feel safe.

3   *Humans are social beings.* Individuals depend on each other to gain support, safety, and for adapting to new and difficult situations. Healthy interactions are our protective factor and as Ludy-Dobson and Perry (2010: 26–27)

say, "the presence of familiar people projecting the social-emotional cues of acceptance, understanding, compassion, and empathy calm the stress response of the individual".

4   *Crisis professionals cannot intervene alone.* In crisis contexts, local actors already exist, and "real help is not that which makes people feel useful, but that which makes local people free and autonomous" (Naiaretti et al., 2009: 17). This approach finds support in the wider concept of "social change".

> Social change is only possible when people in a community have a sense of their own capacity to act, when they become aware of their resources and see themselves as able to re-make the world in which they live. The task of the [play and] expressive arts change agent is not to enter a community with a pre-existing plan, attempting to steer community action in an anticipated direction.
>
> (Levine, 2011: 28)

Play and expressive arts are powerful healing tools (McNiff, 1999; Schaefer and Drewes, 2014) that nonetheless require certain circumstances to be activated. A crisis intervention is not just something to be remembered (in a good or bad way) as an art or play festival, but something tangible that helps to build new possibilities and directions towards an improvement of life conditions. By observing the principles of good practice, many preparatory activities need to be completed. Those that have the greatest chance of being successful in fostering a process of change are those that meet people's need for being accepted, understood, feeling safe, nurtured by healthy relationships, and being actively involved.

Capacity building: more capabilities, opportunities, and choices

People-centred approach offered by the United Nations Development Programme (UNDP) underlines that "human development is about acquiring more capabilities and enjoying more opportunities to use those capabilities. With more capabilities and opportunities, people have more choices" (UNDP, 2016: 25). UNDP conceptualises human development both as a process and as a goal that can be reached by building human resources and by the active engagement of people in the process that impacts and shapes their lives (op. cit.: 2). In the CPBF approach, a training and supervision program can be implemented in collaboration with local partners, only after responding to the primary needs of the crisis. The program is intended for professionals who, most of the time, are *super*vivors (Mochi and Cassina, 2018) or deeply impacted by a critical situation.

We need to explain the term "*super*vivors". We emphasise the precious role that individuals who live in critical conditions and/or survived a disaster might have in managing and overcoming difficulties. The emphasis is on the therapeutic value of the active involvement of individuals who live in critical circumstances and on the scope of their contribution itself. Local professionals and helpers can provide an actual and remarkable contribution by bringing their skills, perspective, and connections to the process.

Focusing on the capacity-building process promotes the effectiveness and sustainability of the work in a crisis. Capacity building allows precious human local resources to develop and strengthen and also enables reach to a larger number of children and families. Not to be underestimated, the aforementioned principles (including respect and "locals know it better") enable the capacity-building process to be enhanced.

The United Nations Academic Impact (2022) defines capacity building as the process of developing and strengthening skills, processes, and resources that an organisation or a community needs. Building people's capacities reflects the flexible and tailored nature of the intervention, and it is rarely completely pre-planned. Initial data for the beginning of the CPBF process are provided by the early assessment, and needs and goals are constantly adjusted on the experience of the activities' implementation and constant relationship with the different actors in the community. The pattern N-G-A offers information and guides the capacity-building process. While we work on meeting a set of identified goals ("coping with the present"), as soon as we detect new needs, we start to get prepared for emerging and more specific needs ("building for the future").

Capacity building is a broad process. The steps we suggest for the capacity-building process are discussed in detail in Chapter 7 and include needs' assessment, training, demonstration and shared activities, observations, supervision, monitoring, new training, and activities.

Applying the therapeutic power of play and play therapy in crisis

The literature includes interesting resources explaining the reasons for using play and play therapy methodologies in crisis (Webb, 1999, 2007; Gil, 2006; Crenshaw et al., 2015). For the purpose of this chapter, it is useful to summarise these reasons as follows (the list has no particular order and cannot be considered exhaustive):

- Play is a universal language and, applied at the ideal time, has the advantage of creating a bridge between people while respecting individuals, communities, and cultures.
- "Children use play to work through and master quite complex psychological difficulties of the past and present" (Bettelheim, 1987). "From a child's play we can gain understanding of how he sees and construes the world – what he would like it to be, what his concerns and problems are" (op. cit.). "Play is [also] the child's most useful tool for preparing himself for the future and its tasks" (op. cit.).
- Play is fundamental for children and adults. Brown (Brown and Vaughan, 2009) argues that play unleashes human potential at every stage of life. Play

"is a crucial dynamic for healthy physical, emotional, behavioural, social and intellectual development at all ages" (Elkind, 2007: 4). It is a source for learning new skills, and it can be useful in fostering personal growth and overcoming psychological problems.

- Play contains all the essential ingredients that foster neuroplasticity (Cozolino, 2010; Wheeler and Dillman Taylor, 2016). In fact, play "promotes consistency and motivation to practice, the creation of a safe environment, the development of trusting relationships, and allows emotional involvement by exposing the player to an ideal level of stimulation" (Mochi and Cassina, 2021: 32).

Figure 1.3 shows the stages of a crisis intervention focusing on the role of play. Through this figure, you will be able to understand why and how play is applied at different moments. Similar to the CPBF chart, there are no deadlines for going from one stage to another, it is a matter of circumstances and perceptions, but each stage is a foundation for the next.

The triangle in the left-hand column in Figure 1.3 reflects the concept of the CPBF chart by including more people in the early stages and then decreasing the number of people as the intervention becomes more specialised. In the initial stage, recreational activities can be implemented to involve as many people as possible. In the advanced stage, psychosocial activities are directed to selected groups of children. In the specialised stage, play therapy interventions involve a small number of children and families who are in need of this kind of involvement.

Starting with recreational activities does not mean that specific treatments are not provided when a clear need is detected. Critical situations may create severe traumatic reactions that require prompt and specialised therapy. For this reason, part of the team should be experienced and prepared to work with people with severe traumatic conditions at any moment. In this regard, it is worth emphasising that the way the three stages are organised (Figure 1.3) and the implementation of the N-G-A pattern underline an important tenet of this process: first identify (assess) and then intervene.

CPBF is also based on the belief that a process of change is more effective when nourished by multiple sources. What happens "outside" the therapy room is at least as important as what happens "inside". Crisis intervention should aim to be a sustainable process in which the individual is not involved in a single therapeutic intervention but in a multitude of positive interactions and healthy activities.

We emphasise that, in order to offer perspective and sustainability to the process, local professionals and helpers must be (as much as possible) in charge of all operations. This means that, in most cases, a certain amount of time is required to build their capacities so that they can respond to emerging needs. The field of goal-oriented play-based activities and play therapy is wide, and the most suitable skills and approaches should be selected and tailored to identified needs (examples are provided in Chapters 3 and 5).

Stage	Objectives	Activities
Initial stage Recreational activities The power of play is used for recreation, connection and assessment.	**Children:** experience a safe context, distraction, fun, release of tension, predictability, socialization with possibility to connect with peers and adults which are active in the project and the community. **Helpers:** involve children in the project. Play helps to build relationships with children and is used as initial identification of psychosocial needs.	Traditional and popular. Lighthearted, fun or sport group activities. Planned and organized by the project team or volunteers. Children can also organize them under team supervision.
Advanced stage Psychosocial activities Play based group activities to promote abilities in children and ameliorate mild psychosocial problems.	**Children:** identification and expression of emotions, self-regulation, coping skills, stress management, etc. **Helpers:** strengthen positive relationships and deeper needs assessment.	Age-specific group activities also extrapolated from different Play Therapy group activities. Each addresses a specific goal. Every session is followed by a report to document the process and results.
Specialized stage Play Therapy Different approaches to prevent or resolve psychosocial problems and psychological disorders and achieve optimal growth and development.	**Children and families:** addressing specific psychosocial needs, post-traumatic or other stress reactions, and multiple problems not improved with psychosocial activities.	Individual, group or family format using Play Therapy methodologies.

Figure 1.3 The stages of a crisis intervention: focusing on the role of play.

Source: Figure reprinted with permission from Beyond the Clouds by Claudio Mochi, copyright (c) 2022 from Loving Healing Press.

Deepen the process through expressive arts

A parallel and complementary process gradually takes more space as the crisis intervention progresses, i.e. the application of play and expressive arts with the goal to support professionals to cope with critical situations. This inclusion in the process brings "the capacity of the arts to respond to human suffering" (Levine and Levine, 1999a: 11), to provide people with possibilities to regain awareness of their own "poietic capacity" (as intended by Levine, 2011: 28) and, by making art, to respond to and shape their world (Knill et al., 2005). More information on the transformative and healing power of play and expressive arts is provided in Chapter 7, including practical examples of how they have been used to overcome critical situations. For the purpose of this chapter, we would like to make clear why we included expressive arts as part of the CPBF crisis intervention process.

Three preliminary considerations are necessary. First, the elements in the CPBF chart are not closed compartments. For example, safety and relationship must be at the centre of our attention all the time, and expressive arts activities and techniques are included from capacity building.

Second, in the academic world, there is more than one opinion on the delineation of the two sectors: play therapy and expressive arts therapy. The two have points in common as well as clear differences. In the play therapy sector, there is wide use of expressive and creative modalities within specific theoretical models (painting and drawing, sand tray and miniatures, writing and storytelling, dramatisation and role-playing, dance and movement, etc.) (Schaefer and Drewes, 2014). On the other side, play is an important component within the expressive arts therapy sector (Levine and Levine, 1999b; Knill et al., 2005; Malchiodi, 2020).

Third, the CPBF chart is not suggesting that play therapy methodologies are used uniquely with children and adolescents. The potential of play and play therapy can be applied in clinical work with adults (Schaefer, 2003). The chart is also not advising that expressive arts therapy and techniques are effective only with adults; they are applied with great benefit to children and adolescents (Malchiodi, 2007). In other words:

> The use of both play and art therapy (the imaginative realm of symbols and image making), with the addition of expressive media such as music, movement, and drama, can provide children and their families and friends [including professionals] with a creative avenue for exploring their worries and psychological suffering induced by traumatic events.
>
> (Gil, Malchiodi and Rubin cited in Byers, 2014: 290–291)

These three considerations are relevant for an overall understanding of the depth of the CPBF process but are not the focus of our chapter. What is important is that the reader is encouraged to think critically and constructively about the chart presented, the potential of play and expressive arts, and the recommended moments for choosing methodologies, techniques, and activities from the two sectors in a crisis context.

The CPBF chart enhances and expands the use of expressive arts with professionals in crisis settings after taking a number of steps. In the CPBF process, the focus gradually shifts from the outside to the inside, or from "caring for others" (i.e. children and families) to "caring for ourselves". Starting the process from here (the "inside") could be overwhelming for participants. The dimensions of play and imagination provide a sense of lightness and fun, but, at the same time, expressive arts can bring out strong and deep emotions, and a safe context must be assured before engaging people with them. The leader (or therapist) is "responsible for maintaining a space of safety and acceptance of individual expression" (Bratton et al., 2014: 261). In the same way, the leader must know the context and the culture well enough to guide the creative experience that could be new and unexpectedly powerful for some participants.

Like a virtuous circle, the playful and creative experience not only has the potential to strengthen professionals personally by encouraging self-awareness, self-expression, and acceptance of self and others, but the more they feel empowered and competent, the more they will be open to new possibilities, including integrating the learnt skills in their work. In fact, for Brown (Brown and Vaughan, 2009: 18), play allows for the realisation of what he calls the "potential for improvisation" through which one's rigidities are overcome and new connections, thoughts, and behaviours are made possible.

Conclusion

The purpose of crisis interventions is to improve the quality of people's lives in the short and long terms. Unfortunately, past events cannot be reversed and some circumstances cannot be modified promptly or at all. That said, the awareness, knowledge, and resources of individuals and support systems can be consolidated and enhanced, which might result in more opportunities and better life conditions.

From the authors' perspective, the capacity-building process is the keystone of crisis interventions as it allows individuals to cope with the present while building for the future. This is true for both individuals (adults and children) and support systems. Crisis professionals have an important role as co-constructors and trainers in the capacity-building process. The therapeutic powers of play and expressive arts are an ideal fit for both adults and children: they open people up to new possibilities, alleviate sufferance, and enable individuals to be authors of their own stories.

If you ever doubt what to do, keep in mind that crisis interventions cannot be "delivered", they need to be co-constructed.

References

Bettelheim, B. (1987) 'The importance of play', *The Atlantic*, 259(3), available: www.theatlantic.com/magazine/archive/1987/03/the-importance-of-play/305129/ [accessed 11 January 2022].

Bratton, S.C., Dillman Taylor, D. and Akay, S. (2014) 'Integrating play and expressive art therapy into small group counseling with preadolescents: A humanistic approach', in E.J., Green and A.A., Drewes (eds.) *Integrating expressive arts and play therapy with children and adolescents*, Hoboken, NJ: Wiley, 253–282.

Brown, S. and Vaughan, C. (2009) *Play: How it shapes the brain, opens the imagination, and invigorates the soul*, New York, NY: Penguin.

Brymer, M., Layne, C., Jacobs, A., Pynoos, R., Ruzek, J., Steinberg, A., Vernberg, E. and Watson, P. (2006) 'Psychological first aid field operations guide', *National Child Traumatic Stress Network*, available: www.nctsn.org/sites/default/files/resources/pfa_field_operations_guide.pdf [accessed 2 October 2021].

Byers, J. (2014) 'Integrating play and expressive art therapy into communities: A multimodal approach', in E.J., Green and A.A., Drewes (eds.) *Integrating expressive arts and play therapy with children and adolescents*, Hoboken, NJ: Wiley, 283–301.

Caplan, G. (1964) *Principles of preventive psychiatry*, New York, NY: Basic Books, Inc.

Carbonnier, G. (2019) 'Revisiting the nexus: Numbers, principles and the issue of social change', *Humanitarian Alternatives*, 10, March 2019, 120–133, available: http://alternatives-humanitaires.org/en/2019/03/25/revisiting-nexus-numbers-principles-issue-social-change/ [accessed 3 December 2021].

Cassina, I. (2009) *Entre l'aide humanitaire et l'aide au développement: La construction d'une cohérence entre principes opposes*, unpublished thesis (M.A.), The Graduate Institute of International and Development Studies in Geneva, Switzerland.

Cozolino, L. (2010) *The neuroscience of psychotherapy: Healing the social brain*, 2nd edn., New York, NY: Norton.

Crenshaw, D.A., Brooks, R. and Goldstein, S. (2015) *Play therapy interventions to enhance resilience*, New York, NY: Guilford Press.

Doherty, G.W. (2007) *Crisis intervention training for disaster workers: An introduction*, Rocky Mountain DMH Institute Press, an imprint of Ann Arbor, MI: Loving Healing Press.

Elkind, D. (2007) *The power of play-how spontaneous, imaginative activities lead to happier, healthier children*, Cambridge, MA: Da Capo Press.

European Civil Protection and Humanitarian Aid Operations (2021) *Forgotten crisis assessment (FCA)*, available: www.dgecho-partners-helpdesk.eu/ngo/financing-decision/dg-echo-strategy/forgotten-crisis [accessed 3 December 2021].

Gil, E. (2006) *Helping abused and traumatized children: Integrating directive and nondirective approaches*, New York, NY: Guilford Press.

Inter-Agency Standing Committee (2007) *IASC guidelines on mental health and psychosocial support in emergency settings*, Geneva: IASC, available: www.humanitarianinfo.org/iasc/content/products [accessed 9 May 2014].

Inter-Agency Standing Committee and the European Commission (2021a) *INFORM report 2021: Shared evidence for managing crises and disasters*, Luxembourg: Publications Office of the European Union, Doi: 10.2760/238523, JRC125620 [accessed 11 December 2021].

Inter-Agency Standing Committee and the European Commission (2021b) *INFORM Risk Index 2022*, Document released 31 August 2021 by the European Commission Joint Research Centre, available: https://drmkc.jrc.ec.europa.eu/inform-index [accessed 4 January 2022].

Joint Research Centre of The European Commission's science and knowledge service (2020) *Humanitarian crises around the world are becoming longer and more complex*, available: https://ec.europa.eu/jrc/en/news/humanitarian-crises-around-world-are-becoming-longer-and-more-complex [accessed 9 December 2021].

Knill, P.J., Levine, E.G. and Levine, S.K. (2005) *Principles and practice of expressive arts therapy. Toward a therapeutic aesthetics*, London: Jessica Kingsley Publishers.

Levine, S.K. (2011) 'Art opens to the world. Expressive arts and social action', in E.G., Levine and S.K., Levine (eds.) *Art in action: Expressive arts therapy and social change*, London: Jessica Kingsley Publishers, 21–30.

Levine, S.K. and Levine, E.G. (1999a) 'Introduction', in S.K., Levine and E.G., Levine (eds.) *Foundations of expressive arts therapy theoretical and clinical perspectives*, London: Jessica Kingsley Publishers, 11–26.

Levine, S.K. and Levine, E.G. (eds.) (1999b) *Foundations of expressive arts therapy theoretical and clinical perspectives*, London: Jessica Kingsley Publishers.

Ludy-Dobson, C.R. and Perry, B.D. (2010) 'The role of healthy interaction in buffering the impact of childhood trauma', in E., Gil, (ed.) *Working with children to heal interpersonal trauma: The power of play*, New York, NY: Guilford Press, 26–43.

Malchiodi, C. (2007) *The art therapy sourcebook*, 2nd edn., New York, NY: McGraw-Hill.

Malchiodi, C. (2020) *Expressive arts therapy and trauma: Using movement, sound, image, and performance to restore the self*, online conference for the United Nations in Geneva, Switzerland, June 2020, available: www.youtube.com/watch?v=SutB72QBvZs [accessed 6 December 2021].

McNiff, S. (1999) 'Artistic inquiry: Research in expressive arts therapy', in S.K., Levine and E.G., Levine (eds.) *Foundations of expressive arts therapy theoretical and clinical perspectives*, London: Jessica Kingsley Publishers, 67–85.

Mochi, C. (2006) *South East Lebanon psychosocial assessment*, Lausanne, Switzerland: Terre des Hommes Foundation for Child Relief.

Mochi, C. (2009) 'Trauma repetition: Intervention in psychological safe places', *Eastern Journal of Psychiatry*, 12(1&2), 75–80.

Mochi, C. (forthcoming 2022) *Beyond the clouds: An autoethnographic research exploring the good practice in crisis settings*, Ann Arbor, MI: Loving Healing Press.

Mochi, C. and Cassina, I. (2018) *Play therapy around the globe: International crisis work with children*, training presented at Northwest Center for Play Therapy Studies Summer Institute, George Fox University, Portland, 6 June 2018.

Mochi, C. and Cassina, I. (2021) *Introduzione alla play therapy. Quando il gioco è la terapia*, Lugano: INA Play Therapy Press.

Mochi, C. and VanFleet, R. (2009) 'Roles play therapist play. Post disaster engagement and empowerment of survivors', *Play Therapy*, 4, December 2009, 16–18.

Naiaretti, C., Sagramoso, A. and Solaro del Borgo, M.A. (2009) *Strumenti operativi per progetti di cooperazione allo sviluppo*, 2nd edn., Lugano: Federazione delle ONG della Svizzera italiana.

Pirotte, C., Husson, B. and Grünewald, F. (2000) *Entre urgence et développement: pratiques humanitaires en questions*, Paris: Karthala.

Porges, S. (2011) *The polyvagal theory: Neurophysiological foundations of emotions, attachment, communication, and self-regulation*, New York, NY: Norton.

Ragaù, S. (2011) *Parola/crisi: Accenni etimologici*, available: https://nonostanterivista.wordpress.com/2011/07/12/parola-crisi-accenni-etimologici-2/ [accessed 15 March 2021].

Schaefer, C.E. (ed.) (2003) *Play therapy with adults*, New York, NJ: Wiley.

Schaefer, C.E. and Drewes, A.A. (2014) *The therapeutic powers of play: 20 core agents of change*, 2nd edn., Hoboken, NJ: Wiley.

United Nations Academic Impact (2022) *Capacity-building*, available: www.un.org/en/academic-impact/capacity-building [accessed 1 January 2022].

United Nations Development Programme (2016) *Human development report 2016: Human development for everyone*, New York, available: http://hdr.undp.org/en/content/human-development-report-2016 [accessed 8 December 2021].

United Nations General Assembly (2017) *Humanitarian crises in Nigeria, Somalia, South Sudan and Yemen*, full transcript of Secretary-General's Joint Press Conference, A/72/1, July 2017, available: www.un.org/sg/en/content/sg/press-encounter/2017-02-22/full-transcript-secretary-generals-joint-press-conference [accessed 4 December 2021].

VanFleet, R. and Mochi, C. (2015) 'Enhancing resilience in play therapy with child and family survivors of mass trauma', in D., Creenshaw, R., Brooks and S., Goldstein (eds.) *Enhancing resilience in play therapy*, New York, NY: Guilford Press, 168–193.

Vocabulary.com (2021) *Crisis*, available: www.vocabulary.com/dictionary/crisis [accessed 20 July 2021].

Webb, N.B. (ed.) (1999) *Play therapy with children in crisis: Individual, group, and family treatment*, 2nd edn., New York, NY: The Guilford Press.

Webb, N.B. (ed.) (2007) *Play therapy with children in crisis: Individual, group, and family treatment*, 3rd edn., New York, NY: The Guilford Press.

Wheeler, N. and Dillman Taylor, D. (2016) 'Integrating interpersonal neurobiology with play therapy', *International Journal of Play Therapy*, 25(1), 24–34.

2 Integrating creative arts modalities in the playroom and outside

Live and remote interventions

Steve Harvey

The use of several creative arts modalities can facilitate therapeutic powers that are part of the natural experience of interactive play that contributes to the individual's development of an alliance, creativity, and an expansion of emotional expression. Mechanisms of change related to the creative arts therapies (CAT) such as active involvement with symbolism, metaphor making, and the enjoyment that accompanies arts-based expression are reviewed. The chapter also addresses how this creative arts/play approach has been applied online with international adult participants in response to the Covid-19 health crisis as well as with families, especially in situations when a verbal understanding is complex.

Russ (1993) has suggested that play can be seen as a process of creative adaption and problem finding/solving to difficulties and challenges that children encounter. Harvey (1994, 2006, 2009) extended this concept to families and suggested that several expressive modalities such as art, dance, drama, and storytelling be integrated within the play action to help family interactions develop more creative adaption to their hardships together. Byers (2014), Harvey and colleagues (Harvey et al., 2018; Harvey et al., 2020b), and Mochi and Cassina (see Chapter 1) describe how expressive arts and play are used to address high distress related to community and international crisis.

McNiff (2004, 2014) states that artistic expression has the unique and timeless ability to touch every person in times of personal crisis and collective distress. Play and the creative/expressive modalities share this unique and timeless ability with artistic expression to help individuals, families, groups, and communities by engaging with underlying creative resources that are integrated using other closely related ingredients of change. Play and other creative expressions both draw on the shared enjoyment and relationship enhancement that emerges from collaborative metaphor making.

Malchiodi and Crenshaw (2014), Gil (2006), Drewes et al. (2011), and Harvey (2016) present a wide range of intervention styles and techniques drawn from both play and the creative arts to address the complex problems that develop with children with trauma and attachment difficulties. In this work, the authors present approaches that incorporate art, drama, dance/movement, and music with play-based action to help families and children develop more

DOI: 10.4324/9781003252375-3

successful communication to develop positive relationship experiences. More recently, Kottman and Meany-Walen (2018: 6) present play therapy as including many types of activities within a therapy setting,

> we would describe play therapy as a therapeutic modality that uses a wide variety of methodologies to communicate with clients, including adventure therapy, storytelling and therapeutic metaphor, music/dance/ experiences, sand tray activities, art techniques, and structured play experiences in addition to free unstructured play.

These authors apply these approaches to individuals, groups, and families of all ages.

In this chapter, I discuss how a generalised approach in which several modalities can be integrated. I then expand on this generalised approach and explain how it can be applied in situations both inside and outside a playroom, online in therapeutic work with children, families, as well as in response to international crisis. The main goal of using several modalities together is to encourage a way for participants to experience new adaptions to the complex dilemmas they encounter using their own creative process.

Dynamic play therapy

Dynamic play therapy (DPT) (Harvey, 1994, 2006, 2009) is an intervention style in which family members are helped to engage in developing play episodes using movement, dramatic storytelling, and artistic expressions together. All family members become included at some time during the intervention, while various parent–child groupings are seen together to develop more specific improvised scenes. The intent of this intervention is to help the family to develop and use the creativity they share among themselves so that they can adapt to their current conflicts with more flexibility and with emotional responsiveness to each other. The central premise is that this creativity is naturally generated to some degree within the context of important basic emotional family relationships and that such creativity is activated in play and other expressive modalities. This natural creativity not only contains problem solving but also facilitates emotional closeness as family members enter, and more fully experience, a state of play with each other.

Russ (1993) reviewed several studies of creativity, play, and affect. She concluded that creativity is associated with more affect-laden thoughts, an openness to affect, and appears to contribute an ability to tolerate and integrate affective material through transformative thought. Further, creativity and creative expressions are associated with the pleasure that comes with problem solving and challenge. Taken together, creativity becomes a central part of understanding how expressive activities contribute to change across many settings. McNiff (2004) stated that creativity is the driving force of change throughout expressive experiences.

Therapeutic powers of play and the creative arts therapies

Schaefer and Drewes (2014) introduced the concept of therapeutic powers that are inherent within play action. These powers are presented as being part of the natural play experience that can be used to design and individualise play intervention for a wide range of situations and contexts. The powers of play are the actual change agents in a play process and connect theory and case formulation to techniques. The therapist can select which powers of play to focus on when considering an approach to develop goals for a client that addresses a complex problem. The general categories of these change agents include facilitating communication, fostering emotional wellbeing, enhancing social relationships, and increasing personal strengths. The specific powers that are generally used to design interventions using the integrations of creative modalities presented in this chapter include the development of the therapeutic alliance, facilitating self-expression, generating positive emotions, developing creative problem solving, enhancement of attachment, and catharsis.

In a similar manner, several international experts in the CAT systematically reviewed a wide range of outcome studies that used CAT (de Witte et al., 2021) to identify the mechanisms of change. The authors summarised change factors that are unique to CAT, especially when the therapies are integrated. These core factors include (1) interventions actively *engage* participants in artistic activity, (2) interventions offer multiple options for both *verbal and nonverbal expression* using *symbolism and metaphor*, (3) interventions facilitate *a process of concretisation to make internal conflicts visible* which enables *perspective taking*, and (4) CATs enhance a sense of creativity and *artistic pleasure* as participants develop some sense of artistic skill in developing expressions related to their personal experiences.

There is considerable overlap between these change elements. Play therapy and CAT modalities contribute to change by facilitating the therapeutic relationship and self-expression and help generate positive emotion, creativity, and catharsis. When the CATs are used within an integrated intervention, the change agents related to these modalities, such as an active use of symbolic and metaphorical communication and creative improvisation, add additional value to the play action.

Overview of integrating play with the creative arts modalities

In work with children and their families who have experienced trauma and disruption, I use methods that are based on attachment and creative process theory (Harvey, 1994, 2006, 2009) and draw on the therapeutic powers that are the most closely related – particularly the development of attachment, expression, positive emotion, and emotional wellbeing. When an integrated approach is being designed to address larger crisis situations, especially in situations outside the playroom, methods are drawn from the theories related to active engagement that involves the collaborative creativity of improvisational metaphor making in addition to methods that address generating emotional safety through attunement. While these problems with families and inter-national crisis are quite different, the principles of engaging participants in actively creating an emotional safety and then co-creating metaphorical and symbolic communication are similar.

These principles have been drawn from the observations of integrated play activities (Harvey, 2006). They highlight how improvisational actions and spontaneity can be developed and integrated together to bring forward expressive interactions. The intention of using these concepts is to guide the emergence of interactive improvisations that are unique to the partici-pants involved and their situation. The interactive improvisations are organ-ised and collaborative and develop a creative experience. The use of several modalities emphasises and extends the experience of this creative process leading to the emergence of complex metaphors that are often quite surpris-ing. These principles also include the development of attuned play, encour-agement of expressive momentum, or a deepening of the engagement of collaborative improvisation, as well as the incorporation of the breaks and deviations in addition to the unexpected and often disturbing emotional expressions that emerge within the play action. This new play action is often surprising and not planned for at the beginning of the process. The creative expressions that emerge for each unique situation are used to develop new metaphor making into a more intimate communication. The concepts and techniques used to integrate play with creative arts modalities are presented in the following.

Attuned play

Attunement within play actions is central for family members or within groups to develop empathy and a joining of emotional states in their com-munication through collaborative creative problem solving. This element is called *attuned play* and is essential to the process. In more physically oriented play, *attuned play* develops as players perform similar actions using the same general expressive rhythms. For example, if a young child begins to use a stop/go pattern of movement within the space, other family members follow using a similar physical pattern that matches at the approximate same speed with the same intention. As play becomes more complicated and dramatic, *attuned play* develops even as players take on actions that require different roles that demand different actions. In *attuned play*, these players develop the same focus on performing a common activity or improvisation. For example, if the players are performing a race, in *attuned play,* they are both trying to win using the same rules. *Attuned play* can become even more complex when players use different play/creative arts modalities such as when one player or set of players are dancing and another player, such as a parent, improvises a story in relation to the action.

Expressive momentum

As attuned play among the players continues independently from an initial structure or therapist directive, the expressive activity can gain a life of its own. Players
become absorbed in their joint action and a play state called *expressive momentum*
develops. As players experience *expressive momentum* together, they become intrinsically engaged, curious, and committed to the experience of the play moment.
Often this is recognised as the "fun" of the play and carries the play action forward
with spontaneity. During *expressive momentum*, collaborative play improvisation has
the feeling that such action can continue indefinitely; in contrast, when this kind
of expression fades, the improvisations become short lived. It is during these times
that the players can develop joint creative leaps that have transformative potential
and find pleasure in each other's initiatives. In the process of *expressive momentum*,
the play process can lead in very surprising directions. *Expressive momentum* is central to generating positive emotion and artistic pleasure and is specifically related to
the experience of playful improvisation. These elements are important ingredients
of change especially as positive emotion emerges. Often moving from one modality to another can extend *expressive momentum*, such as when players co-create a
fairy tale using a drawing or dance they have just completed.

Flow and breaks

The goal of attuned play is for players to develop a flow of expressive momentum in which one play action leads to the next naturally with each player
contributing spontaneously to the overall improvisation independently. Such
improvisation develops a sense of pleasure among the players. However, often,
especially when families have experienced emotional difficulties, breaks to
the attuned play occur as one or several players divert the action by stopping
their contributions as well as the contributions of the other players. Expressive
momentum also stops during these breaks. Breaks can also be more complicated and expressed in the nonverbal communication within play roles. An
example of this kind of situation is when a parent follows a child very closely
while trying to determine the child's free movement stopping the child's movement altogether during a physical game.

Examples of *play breaks* include breaking the pre-established play rules
(implicit as well as explicit), small injuries or aggression (verbal or physical)
towards the play partners when in the play space, stopping and refusing to
continue play action when clear expressive development is available, and/or
strong emotional state changes which are out of context from the play action.
Along with helping to establish attuned play, therapeutic action to redirect
breaks into another style of play flow is an essential intervention to focus the
development of improvisation that can incorporate flow/breaks. The balance
of play flow/break is what leads the therapist's intervention to help the play
action to gain more relevance to the client's unique experience. The breaks in
which a family cannot adapt to themselves with more creative responses and

stop improvisation become a cue for the therapist to include other expressive forms such as moving from a physical game that has stopped to drawing about that experience and then using that drawing to set up a puppet story.

Use of structure and organised activity (form energy balance)

A closely related concept to the use of moment-to-moment play flow and play break is the use of structures to better organise joint expression. This is particularly true when groups of family members are involved. This is called *form/energy balance*. In any improvisational expression, a balance needs to occur in which a general organisation needs to be joined with the energy of spontaneity. When too much form is present, the expressions are meaningless, which consequently loses the interest of the players, and the action will stop. However, when too much energy is present activities can go off in so many directions that the activity loses communicative value. More form is achieved by adding rules, game structures, more defined roles, pre-planning expressive activity, or switching expressive mediums (particularly to art), turn taking, and planning (as with the use of short dramatic scenes). The use of free movement, nondirective play, or simply encouraging what is already occurring, through maximising and extending that expression are ways to help achieve more energy within the play episode. Both structure and expressive energy are required for the ingredients of creativity and positive emotion to emerge from the process of the play actions.

Use of directive and nondirective action

Often the therapist needs to help families or participants in crisis interventions set up initial expressive interactions together so that they can become more able to initially play together with more independence. These activities have a game-like structured interaction with initial roles and turn taking. These games are meant to be an initial starting place for the players to begin improvisations in which there is no set ending or preset objective. Examples include physical activities such as races that can become "slow-motion races", tug of wars, balloon games, and creating drawings or stories using turn taking. Often the therapist can coach the players to begin to include their breaks or other deviations within their interactions so that the beginning game can become an improvised expression that becomes more individualised. It is expected that each of these beginning games will change from the initial structure into something new and evolve to match each individual case situation through play improvisations (Harvey, 1994, 2006).

Core scenes and "hot spots"

As families or community group members begin to use attuned play to improvise with each other, a sense of expressive momentum emerges, and the group can internally find a balance of structure and spontaneity together. Collaborative movement, drama, art, and storytelling can develop into special play scenes that reflect inner emotional states in a metaphorical manner. These metaphors reflect the emotional states not only of an individual but also of a family's or group's emotional environment as well. When this occurs, the therapist identifies and encourages the dramatic themes that emerge into new collaborations. Themes and images, which relate to strong emotions, are particularly relevant, such as anger, loss, death, grief, fear and protection, change, leaving, transition, and (importantly) hope. Such images are considered *hot spots*. Special attention is paid to such images, and they are often creatively elaborated within interventions and extended using other creative modalities. During the working through process of the interventions, the themes and images that emerge are related to significant events, such as episodes of trauma, abandonment, or loss or major concerns for child/family/communities.

Rituals

When specific events are identified, *rituals* can be created to address the very complex emotional responses. The form of these actions is planned by the therapist and family and involves creating symbols from highly emotional scenes that emerged during the intervention. These symbols are co-created using several art modalities and involve art, drama, movement, and storytelling. The events that fit *rituals* include death and loss, family adoption, various goodbyes, change, and ending of therapy.

The play space and resources

To integrate play and create art expression, an expanded use of therapy space is required. In general, this space needs to be larger than is usual in play therapy so that movement and drama are encouraged. There needs to be enough room for full-bodied movement to occur. Props such as scarves, stretch bands, and parachutes are helpful in organising and encouraging movement action as well as physically based imagination. Large pillows are useful to make houses, walls, and props in movement. Toys such as puppets, large soft toy animals, art material, and a sand tray (with figurines) should be available to encourage play and story metaphor. As expressive action develops, therapists can facilitate expressive development from several modalities. Action can move between movement, art, and play easily and/or include all these modes in combination.

When working online, the Zoom screens can be organised in several ways, for example, to isolate the views of various participants to highlight play action into more relevant dramatic conversations. This is reviewed elsewhere (Harvey et al., 2020a).

Metaphorical conversations: an endpoint of the process

One of the main ingredients of change that comes from the integration of play with the creative arts is the communication of nonverbal experience. This is a central goal or endpoint of the process presented earlier. This is the main "working through" portion of the intervention. The client's experiences in this process are highly subjective, related to strong complex feeling, and difficult to communicate verbally. Often these experiences are related to trauma and high distress and can best be expressed through symbolism and metaphor. Rather than trying to reduce these metaphors to verbal concepts, the discussion between family, group members, and the therapist needs to be made within and from the metaphors themselves.

Gil (2014) describes a process of "working the metaphor" in which the therapist considers the products of an expressive process as an externalisation of experiences that cannot be talked about. One goal of the therapist, in talking with the metaphor, is to amplify the aspects of the expression that are often only suggested. The beginning of this process is helping the child/family and adult clients become curious about what has been created in the expression by speaking about and expanding the details without having a preset concept of what it might mean. Often solutions or alternative more positive outcomes emerge from the images in an improvisation. The use of other creative modalities can facilitate this expansion process. For example, a suggested image that arises from a play scene can be expanded using art and then movement.

The important change also occurs when the family or group members are interacting fully and emphatically within the experience of the metaphor. This meeting occurs on several levels (in the experience of play action and within emotional communication) as once the child and family are fully engaged in play, the images are symbolically directly related to important emotional states simultaneously. These moments have been identified as pivotal moments (Harvey, 2011). Such moments of meeting are characterised by an increases in attunement and intersubjective meetings. When such moments occur, the participants can begin to experience their own change with some spontaneity (Ibid.).

McNiff (2014) describes a process in which clients develop a dialogue with the artwork that they have created and encourage these images to creatively speak for themselves. McNiff then describes how other expressive forms such as improvised dance, music, and performance can extend and expand the initial dialogue with the art image. Harvey and Kelly (2018) also described how improvised storytelling and fairy tale making can develop alongside expression from other more nonverbal media such as art and dance. The images and themes that emerge from this creative extension have a transformative quality, a more positive form, and emotional atmosphere and often are quite surprising. These metaphorical conversations are the goal of all the previous techniques (e.g. use of initial starting places, rituals, incorporations of breaks within an expressive flow).

Some initial dance/drama/art structures

Some examples of initial directed activities that lead to the use of several other creativity modalities are presented to illustrate how these initial structures are used to start collaborative improvisation around general themes. It is expected that each starting structure will be transformed through improvisations by the participants to create metaphorical conversations that are relevant to their situation.

The journey/obstacle course

In this activity, the family or group is asked to identify two spots in the room (e.g. a beginning and end of problems). The participants are then coached to use movement to create paths from one spot to another. The participants then select and set up props along these pathways so that the members can move through (such as under with large scarf canopies or parachutes), or over (such as a pile of pillows), or with (such as using pillows or large stuffed animals). Each of these actions can then be identified as being a problem or a strong feeling to facilitate dancing and dramatic action about such concepts. This activity is often used to address the presenting problems, problem solving, or family-related conflicts. The journey can be paired with having the child/family draw a map of the journey prior to or after the journey dance/drama. The child/family can also use the maps or experiences of the journey dance/drama to tell a fairy tale about this journey. This activity can be extended to be used with other family members. This activity can also be used in situations involving community crisis.

The movement scale

This activity expands on feeling scales often used in more cognitive approaches. In the *Movement Scale*, the child and therapist identify a line across the space where one end is an extreme of an emotion (e.g. calm) and the other end is the other extreme (e.g. rage). The child dances the various degrees of the feeling state as he/she moves along the scale from one end or the other. When parent/s participate, the resulting dances can be more directly related to and applied to home activities. Interactions can become playful and creative as caretakers and the child move along the scale. Such movement interaction can also develop relevance in helping the child–parent dyad address the expression, communication, and regulation of strong emotional experiences they have not yet mastered. This activity can be extended by having the child/parent/s/therapist, draw a large version of the scale on a whiteboard prior to the dancing and use the graphic representation to reference the dancing as it is occurring. These drawings should be elaborated in any way according to family wishes to creatively extend the basic scale.

Showing the loudest yell without making a noise

In this activity, the child and adult (parent/caretaker/therapist) are asked to participate in a contest to show the loudest yell without making a noise.

By setting up this task as a competition with roles, each participant can be encouraged to use their body more completely while making playful non-verbal conversations. The activity can be extended by selecting different body parts to be used, such as a face or feet, and how quickly or slowly the moment can be done. The child and parent can then be asked to creatively extend their movement into dancing based on these themes. Art activities are used alongside these dances to express various feelings. The goal of the task is to have the child and important adult/s develop nonverbal exchanges using dance with emotions as the basic theme. Storytelling can be added to expand on the dance and/or drawing creation about the interactive actions that express externalisation of experiences that cannot be talked about. One goal in talking with the metaphor is to amplify the aspects of the expression that are often only suggested. The beginning of this process is helping the child/family and adult clients become curious about each other's expressions beyond their usual interactions and then how such new expressions can be joined together.

Application of creative arts therapies in a complex world

DPT (Harvey, 1994, 2006, 2009) was initially developed as a family therapy process to work with children and families who had experienced significant attachment and traumatic experiences together. Several of the children were in a government child protective service due to various forms of significant abuse from within their families. The creative play process of DPT has been expanded and applied to other problem contexts such as responses to incidents that involve social trauma (Harvey and Kelly, 2020a, 2020b) and political tension across countries (Harvey et al., 2018). Most recently, this style of integrated creative expression has been applied to adults from several countries and cultures via Zoom to address the distress that has come with the Covid-19 pandemic (Harvey et al., 2020a; Harvey et al., 2020b; Harvey and Wang, 2022).

The common theme, when working across these complex areas, is that underlying problems are too complex to be placed solely in a verbal context. In these events, people's subjective emotional experience can involve multiple responses to the event/s at the same time. Often these feelings are conflicting and are not resolved easily alongside high levels of distress. Also, people often experience high degrees of internal and social/family conflict in addition to their difficult inner states. Children do not have the verbal maturity to easily understand, express, or participate in the verbal processing of such complex events. Families can become helpless when they experience trauma, especially when parents cannot communicate effectively with their children. Collaborative metaphor making can help address these situations nonverbally as complex subjective experience can be expressed within images and arts-based metaphors. This use of metaphor making can engage children within an intervention when it is important to involve them. While children can be left out of and have difficulty in offering a meaningful role in the verbal discussion, they can participate more fully in co-creating play expressions such as those presented.

Community crisis situations may also have emotionally related elements that can benefit from more nonverbal and arts-based metaphor making. As creative metaphorical communication among the participants develops in a meaningful way, further discussion can become refocused on relevant personal emotional experiences in contrast to verbal consideration which can become saturated with conflict and complexity. Community events can become embedded within significant conflict and political tension, which typically involve verbal contexts that reflect and amply the conflict. Often community-based verbal communication hinders the understanding and successful coping or processing of subjective and emotional experiences of individuals or small groups. Examples of interventions with both family and community-based events will be presented to illustrate how creative art applications can add an important part of a resolution to conflict.

CASE EXAMPLES

Case study 1. Family sessions: finding attachment in an unreasonable world

The following case is a fictionalised composite account. While this case does not reflect specific clinical details, it does represent themes and events that have occurred.

Emma, an 8-year-old girl, was referred by her mother when she began to run into the street saying that she wanted to end her life. During the intake interview, her mother, Janice, reported that Emma was unable to sleep, often wet the bed, had periods of nonstop crying, and was becoming inconsolable when she returned from her father's home after visits. At school, Emma had become very impulsive in class and was aggressive to her peers to the point that she was often required to return home. Janice provided a social, family, educational, and history of trauma.

When Emma was 5, a relative reported that she had observed Emma's father engaged in what appeared to be a sexual act while he was taking care of her. This event led to a divorce and legal proceedings in which it was alleged that Emma's father had sexually assaulted her. An evaluating psychologist determined that the relative was an unreliable witness and had influenced Emma's statements in later interviews with police and the child protective services. A judge determined that no sexual assault had occurred, and he ordered Emma to continue to have access to her father. Joint custody was set up. Janice reported that she brought her daughter to a mental health service at the time of the trial with similar behaviours related to emotional dysregulation. Emma had been provided with a short-term course of non-directive play therapy, which had helped reduce her more impulsive behaviours; however, the family conflict was not addressed. These highly dysregulated behaviours returned as overnight visitations with her father increased.

The therapist suggested that the therapy uses expressive modalities and initially addresses Emma's impulsive extreme emotional expressions and more dangerous behaviours such as running into the street, as well as improves Emma and Janice's relationship. The therapist and Janice agreed that expressive play collaborations with her would be important as it was essential for Emma to become actively involved in developing more control over her behaviour and she was unlikely to accomplish this using verbal conversations. It was also agreed that the distress coming from the extended family's ongoing conflict was highly complex and could not be effectively addressed verbally in the therapy setting as the verbal narratives had too many conflicting versions. The therapist suggested that Janice and Emma begin using interactive expressive play as the primary activity.

After the intake interview, the therapist set up several sessions for conjoint play using movement, art/story making, and dramatic enactment together. Emma and Janice began by improvising a game of following the leader with both having a turn to be the leader. During this action, Emma kept disrupting any joint play activity with her impulsivity. She would not let Janice develop leadership. The game ended quickly leaving both mother and daughter feeling frustrated and irritated. Emma and her mother were then asked to make a story about a family using large stuffed animals and pillows. Emma became intent on knocking the animals and pillows over as they were being set up by Janice. Again, this activity was over quickly and was unsatisfying for the participants. In the last part of the session, Emma and Janice were asked to take turns to develop a drawing story by creating a village and then show themselves interacting. Emma dominated the expression by drawing herself in a house that soon become engulfed in a large fire. When this developed, the therapist helped guide Janice to draw rescue equipment and draw herself rescuing Emma. The story was finally a way that Janice and Emma could become more collaborative.

In the next meeting, the therapist helped Janice consider how (1) Emma had played, (2) the images that emerged related to her daughter's problems with high emotion, and (3) her behavioural intensity, especially during interactions. The therapist and Janice also considered the need to develop more form or structure within their expression to generate more expressive momentum or interest for positive emotion to emerge. The experience of unresolved family conflict as well as the possible actual experience of assault was still highly distressing, had impacted the feelings for attachment security, and created a mismatching and breaks within the nonverbal attunement between Janice and Emma. The play action of the treatment was represented to Emma as play to help develop a rescue from the fires. The therapeutic powers of expression, development of positive emotion, and enhancement of attachment, along with possible catharsis that might come from play action, would help in the design of the expressive activity. The development of active engagement in metaphorical conversations in whatever form they emerged would provide additional potential for change.

During the next several sessions, structured movement and art activity were directed by the therapist. The therapist helped Emma develop a movement scale of an increasing intensity of feeling from calm to "wild" across the open space. Emma identified the calm end as a calm lake. The spaces for steps of increased intensity were labelled as the burning sun, fire, forest fire, to the extreme end as roaring fire. Emma then developed movement responses at each level. She used the "scream as loud as you can without making a sound" to structure her movement. Emma and Janice then made art to express each level. Emma and Janice then made dances together during the next session to express different types of intensity. The use of silent movement helped Emma develop a form that included more expressive and longer movement phrases. Janice was coached to respond to this movement in an attuned way to create duets together with Emma. Emma became excited to teach her mother her "dance feelings".

After this series of activities, Emma and Janice were asked to create a life size body drawing of Emma. Emma was then asked to use all the colours to fill the inside of this body outline with her feelings in the part of her body that she experienced them. Emma was able to use this body drawing to then respond with her body. Janice and Emma were able to use dancing to tell stories about different characters and the feelings from within the body drawing. Janice and Emma took this drawing home and put it in a place where each could refer to it and continue this story making. Emma and her mother then created a book illustrated with their art in session, telling their favourite fairy tales.

Both Emma and Janice reported that their relationship improved soon after these collaborations. Emma had stopped trying to run into the street, saying she wanted to end her life, and her behaviour at school improved to the point she was not being asked to stay home. However, she continued to have sleep difficulties with upsetting dreams. Janice, Emma, and the therapist decided that Emma would have some individual sessions in which she could develop her own stories. During these individual sessions, Emma chose to make sand trays and art to elaborate the characters and plot. These trays became dramatic. Themes emerged in which much larger animals overwhelmed a small figure. Emma often buried the small figure to protect her. In the drawings, the larger figures became extremely dangerous and all powerful. At this point, the therapist and Emma decided to invite Janice into the play to help. As the play developed into a more full-bodied drama, this series of sessions ended with Janice designing a fortress with life-sized large walls for her and Emma to live in.

The intervention ended soon after this development. Many of Emma's problems had been resolved. Both Janice and Emma reported that their relationship had improved, and both reported that the "most terrible fires" had receded. The last few sessions were devoted to planning the ritual to mark the ending of therapy. The therapist, Emma, and Janice used artwork and writing to create a large card to exchange with the therapist as presents at the last session.

Art was based on the most important memories each had during the session. These images included representations of the body drawing full of feelings and the stories that came from this, the walls that marked the safe territory of the playroom, and the dance of the silent yelling that came from the roaring fire.

During the individual sessions, Emma did make additional reports about her father's sexual approaches to her. These reports were forwarded to the relevant legal and child protective agencies involved. Emma's accounts were determined to be credible by these agencies. However, in the court action, the judge upheld the earlier decisions that these statements were not credible and joint custody continued. Therapy ended with these legal conflicts largely unresolved. However, despite this inconclusiveness, Emma and Janice were able to describe how their emotional lives together had changed.

Case study 2. Creative dialogues: an arts-based international online project during Covid-19

The international health crisis of the Covid-19 pandemic changed community life across the world in many ways from the smaller more practical details related to travel and social restrictions to the larger issues of the emotional climate during times of distress, tragedy, and death. The national and international political conflicts added the potential for misunderstanding among countries and within communities. Social and political commentary dominated much of the public dialogue and often added more community conflict, leaving few avenues for expression and communication of personal emotional experiences with each other. The Creative Dialogues project is an international project that began with the earliest part of the pandemic to address this gap. As of this writing, this project is ongoing.

The project began as an experiment with no expectation as to what would develop. The initial meeting was set up between a small group of creative arts therapists from China, Guam, and the USA as an online forum in late January 2020 when the health crisis was emerging in China (Harvey et al., 2020b). The group's intention was to investigate if we could develop empathic communication of the subjective experience with our Chinese colleagues online. We had no plan beyond this experiment, and our goal was to develop an avenue for an experience of shared empathy and goodwill with those in the East using the creative arts. The central point was to follow what emerged from our session. As the pandemic spread across the world, we expanded the project to include people in other countries to use creative exchange to develop metaphors with each other. During our experiences, we have found that our structures and expressions have been evolving through group improvisations to match our ongoing experiences.

This project has developed to include small groups of adults from several parts of the world who meet online and use improvisational creative arts to communicate personal experiences of the health crisis with each other. Often the participants do not have a common primary language. One of the early discoveries was that intimate communication, attunement, and empathy could develop online (Harvey et al., 2020b), alongside the emergence of a spontaneous collaborative creative process around themes, metaphors, and images of personal experience (Harvey and Wang, 2022). These shared group creative experiences appear to contribute to the development of community resilience and reduce common experiences of alienation from our communities as the social media and political leaders began to introduce divisive public expression.

The online Zoom groups in this project consisted of five to ten participants from different countries. Some participants have an interest in the creative arts, while others do not. Each group member participates in each session using improvisational dance, art, music, poetry, and story making followed by conversations about their experiences. The improvisations began with some structure related to the personal experiences of group members. The group has a leader trained in CAT and play therapy.

One of the structured starting places is organised with a participant telling a personal account of an experience with the pandemic and then choosing a participant from another country to improvise a short dance using their current physical experience after hearing the story, rather than trying to create a concrete mime of the initial story. Musician/s join the dancer to create an improvised duet. The musician/s and dancer collaborate by following each other's expressions with attunement to each other and without a pre-set choreography or ending. As the virus was moving across the world, a trio form has developed. In this structure, each dancer responds to the other dancers within their improvisation. Musicians also joined this performance. Occasionally, musicians improvise duets without movers. The final structure of each session is set up with a dancer/s improvising movement in collaboration and in response to other group members who improvised a fairy tale as they watched the emerging movement and vocalisation. It is assumed that the dance/music/improvised story in concert with the audience's active imagination will contain a summary of the imagery and themes of the central emotional experiences that have emerged creatively and in imaginary ways during the session. As the project has developed, we often add two languages (English and Mandarin, for example) within the fairy tale.

Group participants respond to the episodes with spontaneous art and poetry making to extend the metaphors using other modalities. As they witness the performances, the watching group members use their active imagination in creating these art-based responses. The watchers are far more active than is typical within groups and are considered full partners in expressive collaborations. These improvisations are designed to develop an attuned expression that can develop expressive momentum through collaborations. Often each episode stimulates the following stories to develop metaphorical conversations that have more meaning in surprising ways.

A series of pictures from dance improvisation, art/poetry responses, and the fairy tale developed from these expressions is presented to illustrate the development of metaphorical conversation with an online group. These examples are from a session during the home lockdown from the initial wave of infections within the countries of the participants in April 2020. Participants were from China, Guam, and Australia in this session.

The initial stories from this session related to the frustrations and loneliness coming out of the social distancing and restrictions on contact with family that many of the participants were experiencing. Several group members told of sadness of having neighbours physically distancing from them on the street, having a meeting with a new grandchild on Zoom and not being able to touch or hold them, and staying at a distance from a group of close friends in a regular gathering. Some of the participants told these stories and then selected another participant from another country to create a dance improvisation. Some of these stories and the art responses are illustrated in the following.

After the dance, the woman who presented this story said that she realised that the meeting with her grandchild was one-sided because the infant could not respond back online. From her image of the dance (see Figure 2.1), she reported that the online meeting felt like looking into a grey screen and devoid of the feeling of an important relationship.

The participant who had presented the story of how stressful a meeting with her friends had been after they were going into their initial social restrictions remarked that the dance helped her realise just how much fear and uncertainty she was experiencing as she was not able to move closer to her friends (see Figure 2.2).

Following these episodes, one participant presented a story of how she had started to care for a family member's pet turtle while her relative was away. She related that this was one of the few contacts she was able to have during this time as she was living alone. She reported her feeling of developing some closeness with this "living being", the turtle. The group leader presented this dance as "a different kind of love affair".

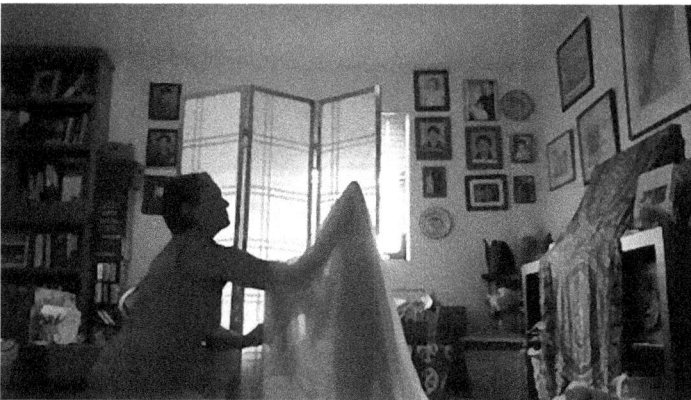

Figure 2.1 A dance improvisation of meeting family on Zoom.

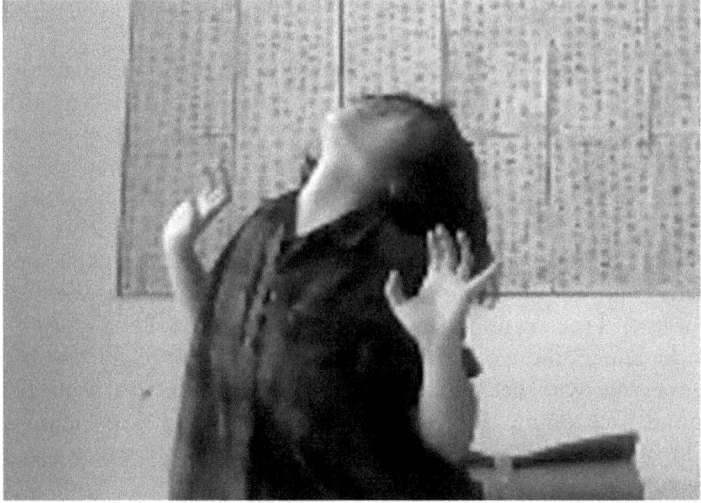

Figure 2.2 An improvisation of meeting good friends with social distance.

A dancer from another country was selected. The dance improvisation was short and used circular shapes and a reaching towards and away from the dancer's body. After the dancer completed her dance, she said she not only felt that she had the feeling of wanting to connect coming from inside her body, but also felt great uncertainty (see Figures 2.3 and 2.4). She continued by saying that in the dance she had become both a person and a turtle living in the same world, "we are each other".

Following the improvisation, the dancer created an art piece that had a purple circle in the middle of a large oval of other colours. She reported that "each person has energy inside their body, and we need to find it and have it spread out" (see Figure 2.5).

Poetry response to the dance

The woman who created this piece was from China. She told of how in ancient Chinese stories that four turtles carry the earth on their backs. The art is of a turtle. Her poem:

The earth is asleep waiting to wake up.

Another woman in the group presented this poem. Her art was of a very light line that crossed from the bottom to the top.

The shell falls away. A shell I didn't even know was there.
Drifting up like smoke into the sky following the wind.

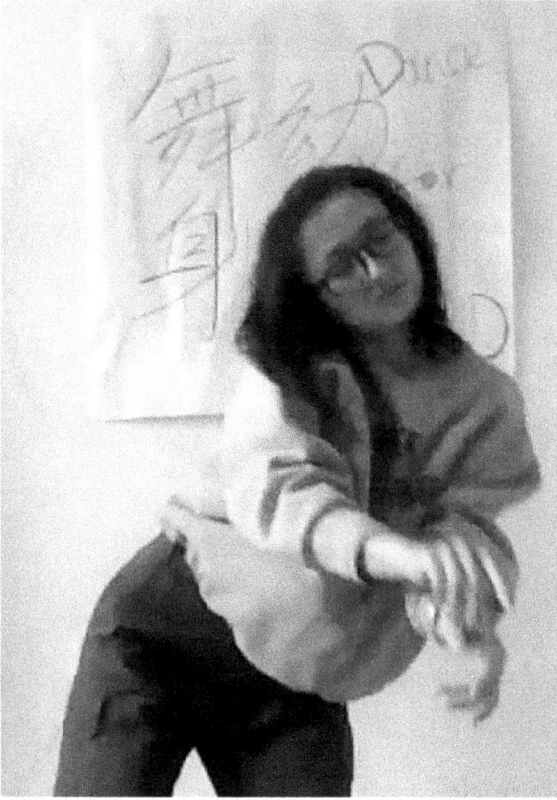

Figure 2.3 The dance of "A different kind of love affair".

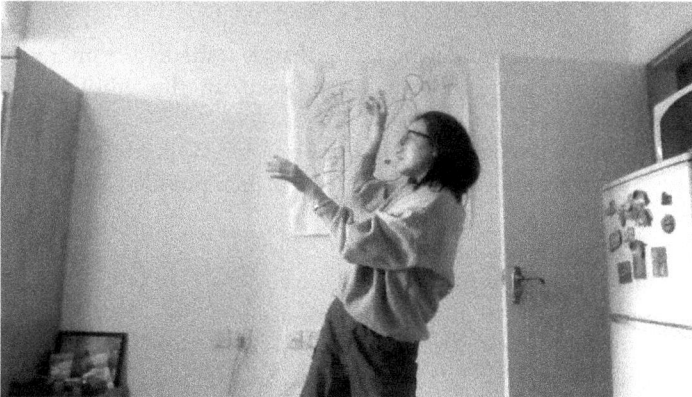

Figure 2.4 The dance of "A different kind of love affair".

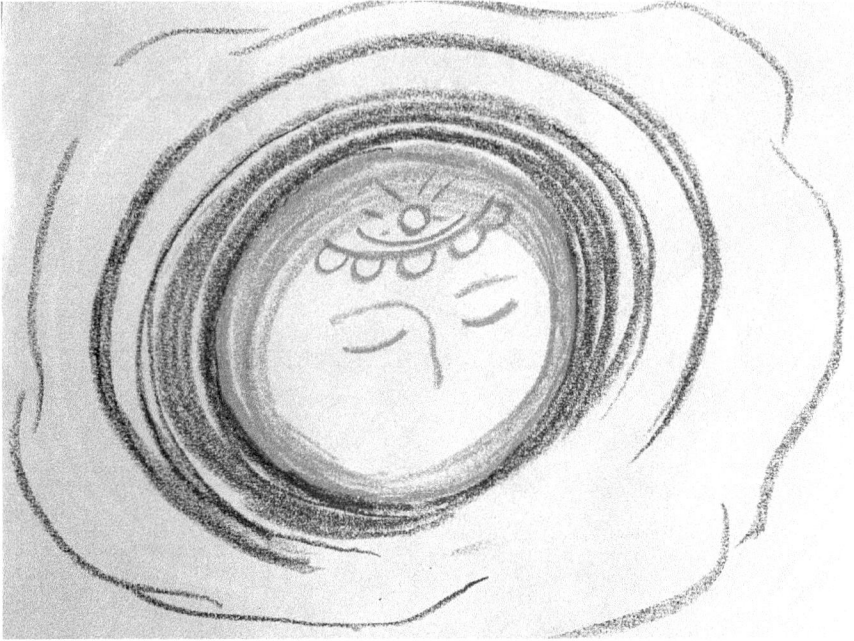

Figure 2.5 Drawing from the dance of "A different kind of love affair".

The summary fairy tale

At the end of session, one dancer improvised movement, while another impro-vised a fairy tale together. This was not pre-set, and neither participant knew the direction the image might take or how it would end. The fairy tale was seen as a summary of themes generated in the session (see Figure 2.6).

> When the sun was considering rising that day/she had many reservations.
> "It is an exhausting job actually to wake up the whole world", she thought.
> "Can't I just wait and put everything on hold? Well, not really".
> Because deep inside of her/Very deep in her muscles/Very deep in her nerves/
> And her blood circulation,
> She kept reaching and reaching,
> And the day began.
> Once she was above the clouds/The dance could be seen and felt everywhere.
> "Come let me bring you the day in warmth and in light.
> Because I am here, and you are here".

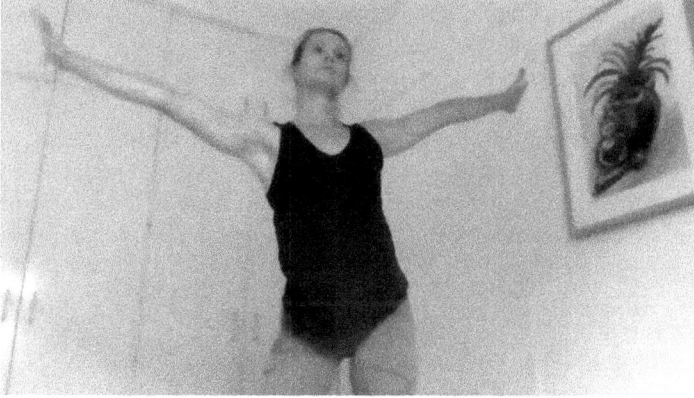

Figure 2.6 The dance of the sunrise: a fairy tale.

During this session, the distress, fear of the virus, and uncertainty the group felt during the beginning restrictions was expressed in discussions. Social restrictions and isolation of the global health crisis were then actively addressed in the initial shared creative expression. The group developed extended metaphors around each story of a personal experience. The collaborative creative process became transformative. A communication developed around emotional experiences that were important for our group members. A sense of empathic connection emerged. This was not expected and was a surprise. Importantly, the group was able to generate a strong positive emotional tone with each other using creative collaborations as the session progressed. The imagery changed dramatically from expressing a sense of isolation and distress to a shared experience of reaching out for emotional connection in the metaphorical conversation. The images created throughout the session culminating with the fairy tale point to a coherence and meaning around a theme of hope and possibility of positive social connection. This feeling tone contributed to a sense of a possible future despite the initial distress. Each of the group members said this helped them feel a sense of community that had been significantly challenged.

Conclusion

Creative arts/play therapies have much to contribute when events are too complex to fit within a verbal context. Times of crisis when families and communities experience high distress, trauma, and several simultaneous emotional states are often accompanied by social conflict. Verbal communication can become overwhelming and inadequate and can lead to significant isolation when intimate communication is needed most in situations of social, legal, and political conflict. The process of making collaborations using the creative arts offers avenues to actively engage families and communities in communicating through symbolism and metaphor with each other. The experiences of meeting within these metaphorical conversations do help participants change and re-focus communications towards intimacy.

This chapter has presented an approach to using several creative modalities including play that have been integrated to expand collaborative metaphor making among families and small groups. The central premise of the integration is based on the idea of activating the change agents from both play therapies and the CAT. The goal of this integration is to facilitate an extended process in which participants can actively construct a complex expression that matches their inner experiences and make moments of intimate meeting that bring the experience, the pleasure, and the shared positive feeling that comes with co-creativity.

Both case examples presented occurred within ongoing social conflicts and in combination with high levels of internally felt distress. The mother and daughter came to therapy while a legal proceeding concerning custody/visitation and allegations of sexual misuse were ongoing with all indications it would continue without resolution or adequate verbal definition. During the Creative Dialogue groups, the pandemic health crisis was occurring bringing conflicts related to the social restrictions and political tensions within and between countries at a time when death rates continued to increase. However, in both these examples, the participants were able to develop intimate communication with each other using creative and playful collaborations. When the mother and her daughter, and the Creative Dialogue group members began to meet, they were expressing inner distress and the negative influences such as alienation from their social circumstances. As they were able to actively engage with each other in creating metaphors about their personal experience, they began to develop a shared inner focus that led to a positive change.

References

Byers, J. (2014) 'Integrating play and expressive art therapy into communities: A multimodal approach', in C.A., Malchiodi and D.A., Crenshaw (eds.) *Creative arts and play therapy for attachment problems*, New York, NY: The Guilford Press, 283–303.

de Witte, M., Orkibi, H., Zarate, R., Kartov, V., Malhorta, B., Ho, R., Baker, E. and Koch, S. (2021) 'From therapeutic factors to mechanisms of change in the creative arts therapies', *Frontiers in Psychology, Open-Source Journal*, 12, 1–27, Doi: 10.3389/fpsyg.2021.678397.

Drewes, A.A., Bratton, S.C. and Schaefer, C.E. (2011) *Integrative play therapy*, Hoboken, New Jersey: Wiley & Sons.

Gill, E. (2006) *Helping abused and traumatized children: Integrating directive and nondirective approaches*, New York, NY: The Guilford Press.

Gill, E. (2014) 'The creative use of metaphor in art and play therapy with attachment problems', in C.A., Malchiodi and D.A., Crenshaw (eds.) *Creative arts and play therapy for attachment problems*, New York, NY: The Guilford Press, 159–178.

Harvey, S.A. (1994) 'Dynamic play therapy: Expressive play interventions with families', in K.J., O'Connor and C.E., Schaefer (eds.) *Handbook of play therapy: Volume two advances and innovations*, Hoboken, New Jersey: Wiley & Sons, 85–111.

Harvey, S.A. (2006) 'Dynamic play therapy', in C.E., Schaefer and H., Kudson (eds.) *Contemporary play therapy*, New York, NY: The Guilford Press, 55–81.

Harvey, S.A. (2009) 'Family problem solving', in A.A., Drewes, (ed.) *Blending play therapy with cognitive behavioural therapy: Evidence based and other effective treatment and techniques*, Hoboken, New Jersey: Wiley & Sons, 449–470.

Harvey, S.A. (2011) 'Pivotal moments of change in expressive therapy with children', *British Journal of Play Therapy*, 7, 74–85.

Harvey, S.A. (2016) 'Using drama in play therapy'', in C.E., Schaefer and L.D., Braverman (eds.) *Handbook of play therapy*, 2nd edn., Hoboken, New Jersey: Wiley & Sons, 289–308.

Harvey, S.A. and Kelly, E.C. (2018) 'Investigating the fairy-tale score used in physical storytelling', *Moving On*, 15, Dance Therapy Association of Australasia, 2–12.

Harvey, S.A. and Kelly, E.C. (2020a) 'Investigating the solo score used in physical storytelling', *Moving On*, 17–18, 32–41, Dance Therapy Association of Australasia.

Harvey, S.A. and Kelly, E.C. (2020b) 'Physical storytelling as modern ritual for political conflict', *Moving On*, 17–18, 42–50, Dance Therapy Association of Australasia.

Harvey, S.A., Kelly, E.C. and Jennings, C. (2020a) 'Creative dialogues across countries: Towards modern performance online during the global health crisis related to COVID 19', *Drama Therapy Review*, 6(2), 1–6.

Harvey, S.A. and Wang, B. (2022) 'Creative arts online: Connection when physical presence is not possible'', *Moving On*, 18(1,2), 3–21.

Harvey, S.A., Wang, S., Kelly, E.C., Wittig, J., Li, X., Peng, X. and Tingting, S. (2020b) 'Creative dialogues across countries and culture during COVID 19', *Creative Arts in Education and Therapy*, 6(1), 74–84, Doi: 10.15212/CAET/2020/6/13.

Harvey, S.A., Zhou, T., Kelly, E.C. and Wittig, J. (2018) 'Physical conversations between the east and west: An arts-based inquiry into the cross-cultural emotional climate during a time of political tensions', *Creative Arts in Education and Therapy*, 4, 1–20.

Kottman, T. and Meany-Walen, K. (2018) *Doing play therapy: Form building relationship to facilitating change*, New York, NY: The Guilford Press.

Malchiodi, C.A. and Crenshaw, D.A. (2014) *Creative arts and play therapy for attachment problems*, New York, NY: The Guilford Press.

McNiff, S. (2004) *Art heals: How creativity cues the soul*, London: Shambala.

McNiff, S. (2014) *Art as medicine: Creating a therapy of the imagination*, Boulder, Co: Shambala Publications.

Russ, S.W. (1993) *Affect and creativity: The roles of affect and play in the creative process*. Hillsdale, NJ: Lawrence Erlbaum Associates.

Schaefer, C.E. and Drewes, A.A. (2014) *The therapeutic powers of play: 20 Core agent of change*, Hoboken, NJ: Wiley & Sons.

3 Recovering lost play time

Principles and intervention modalities to address the psychosocial wellbeing of asylum seekers and refugee children

Isabella Cassina

The chapter is written from the perspective of a professional providing psychosocial support to children showing aggressiveness, lack of self-control and social competences, depression, anxiety, low self-esteem, hyperactivity, and developmental issues. The questions addressed in this chapter are: what do displaced children need most once they reach our service? How do we involve their families in the process? Why, when, and how do we introduce and use the therapeutic power of play and, more specifically, play therapy interventions?

The answers to these questions unfold throughout the chapter by providing a theoretical orientation on children's psychosocial needs, a concrete example of a project developed in a reception centre by the author and her team, and a case study with a child in child-centred play therapy (CCPT).

In 2006, I was in Colombia for my first humanitarian work experience. By then, I had decided to specialise with a master's degree in International and Development Studies. In 2010, I started my Play Therapy training program, when I was already working in Serbia for a local non-governmental organisation. A few months later, I moved back to Switzerland and I obtained a job with a major humanitarian organisation in the role of social worker and head of social services of reception centres for asylum seekers and refugees.[1]

The main centre I worked in hosted up to 120 guests, most of them were families with children aged 0–12 years. Depending on the international migration flow, sometimes more than 30 different nationalities lived under the same roof. As a social worker, I was able to listen to life stories, hopes, and fears. During the first couple of years, most of the work my colleagues and I did was to support and guide adults in a new and temporary routine (looking for a short-term job, learning Italian, dealing with administrative and medical procedures, etc.). Children were enrolled in school and occasionally referred to an external mental health service. Our office was open daily, and we shared with most of the guests moments of joy and sadness, we listened to concerns about family members, past misadventures, the frustration of waiting for an answer to the asylum application, and the fear of being removed from Switzerland. Over time, I was more and more aware of the impact that forced displacement had, especially on children's psychosocial wellbeing and how much more we could

DOI: 10.4324/9781003252375-4

do to improve our support to families during their stay in the centre. This is what this chapter is about.[2]

The process of migration and the Avalanche Metaphor

The definition of migration is "the movement of persons away from their place of usual residence, either across an international border or within a State" (International Organization for Migration IOM, 2021). My work experience has taught me that migration is a process that does not start when people leave a country, nor does it end once they have reached a new one where they ask for asylum. As much as this may seem contradictory to the original definition, it gives us a better perspective of the roots and how massive the psychosocial consequences are of migration, particularly forced migration. The response to this phenomenon needs to be specific and effective.

From this perspective, we can detect three main moments in the migration process (Cassina and Mochi, 2017). The first is *before the travel*, and it can last for years. Before leaving one's country, people might have lived for a long time in very difficult psychosocial conditions generated and nourished by violence, neglect, poverty, exclusion and discrimination, natural disasters, internal conflicts, and war. The second moment is the *travel*, the change to one or more locations which is sometimes considered migration itself. This displacement leads migrant families to the country where they ask for asylum. This period too can last for years, and many times it is characterised by the neglect of primary needs, physical abuse and exploitation, lack of reference points and unpredictability, separation from family members, poor hygienic conditions, health issues, and diseases. The third moment is *after the travel*, which is basically when we meet the families in the service I worked for.

The third moment, *after the travel*, presents new complexities for people as each country has its own social system and deals differently with the care of migrant children and parents (a term that should always be understood in this chapter as caregivers as well). For child professionals, it is easy to understand that difficulties do not end all of a sudden *after the travel*, but rather, new ones can arise: migrants might have to deal with an unknown language, significant cultural differences, unfavourable economic situation, critical medical and psychological conditions, exclusion and poor socialisation possibilities, and uncertainty about the future, to name a few.

That said, let's focus on children. I saw hundreds of minors in my work who had faced years (sometimes since they were born) of an increasing and accumulating number of difficulties that persisted once they reached Switzerland. The children presented with conditions such as aggressiveness, confusion, sadness, lack of self-control and social competences, depression, anxiety, high levels of stress, low self-esteem, developmental issues and physical discomfort, hyperactivity, and a persistent state of fear. Such conditions, especially when they are carried for a long period of time, exacerbate the vulnerability of children, can be traumatic, and deprive them of the experiences necessary for their growth, especially of the possibility to play, which is the most natural and dynamic self-healing process in which children can engage (Erikson, 1950). Considering the condition of stress, fear, uncertainty, and sometimes trauma that weighs on parents, for many children, migration takes place with a progressive accumulation of risk factors and a drastic reduction of protection factors.

In this regard, I find it appropriate to introduce The Avalanche Metaphor (Cassina, 2019) to fix the main idea behind the migration process as described so far. "An avalanche is typically triggered when material on a slope breaks loose from its surroundings; this material then quickly collects and carries additional material down the slope" (Encyclopædia Britannica, Inc., 2021). In the same way as it happens for the avalanche, the difficulties arising from the migration process accumulate over time and the whole enlarges and consolidates. "The occurrence of an avalanche depends on the interaction of mountainous terrain, weather conditions, snowpack conditions, and a trigger", but "certain types of weather lead directly to dangerous avalanche conditions" (op. cit.). In migration, children encounter objective difficult conditions and sometimes they face a trigger too, a striking event that overwhelms them completely and starts them on a fast descent. We cannot state that all migrants suffer from post-traumatic stress disorder, because life stories are various and everyone reacts differently to the situations they encounter. Nevertheless, in the period of time that starts from the life in the country of origin, the travel through one or more countries of transit, and the arrival to the country of destination, we can assume that children experience unfavourable conditions for their development and wellbeing. Moreover, "every experience that exceeds their control and their capacity to cope is anxiety provoking and potentially traumatizing" and "no one is to be considered immune from the occurrence of psychological symptoms in the aftermath of a critical event" (Webb, 2007: 6–7). One last aspect of the Avalanche Metaphor introduces the role of child professionals. "In order to reduce fatalities and to protect villages and roads, people attempt to predict and prevent avalanches. . . . In addition to predicting avalanches, people employ a variety of techniques to reduce avalanche danger" (Encyclopædia Britannica, Inc., 2021). As child professionals, we cannot stop avalanches from happening, but we can create the conditions to stop them from getting bigger, and, with the right amount of therapeutic skill and time, we can have a significant role in dissolving them and repairing its disasters.

As Perry (2005) points out, exposure to high and constant stress levels can arrest the child in a state of attack or flight by permanently altering his neural systems, and, according to Goleman (1997), this can create deficits in intellectual ability that impair children's learning. Children learn through play, and play is the language of children, their natural means of expression (Landreth, 2002), as well as the most natural and dynamic process of self-healing. In the process of migration, children's ability, inclination, and concrete possibility to play can be very limited or nil. A child's lack of access to play and play resources has challenging consequences for a child's development and wellbeing (Brown and Vaughan, 2009) and is the primary reason why play must be part of the healing process and children sustained in expanding and affirming this precious inclination. A prompt and timely intervention from child professionals in the country of destination allows children to start recovering the play time they lost, and through play, recovering from complex psychosocial conditions. This brings us to the concept of "Recovering lost play time" (Cassina, 2015) which is at the heart of children's issues in the migration process (but it is not limited to it) and the response that professionals can provide. "Recovering lost play time" is exactly what my colleagues and I started implementing systematically in the centre we worked in.

More than once people from outside the reception centre told me: "They are safe now, no more violence nor war, they don't have to worry about food nor money, children go to school and have toys, isn't this enough?". It depends, enough for who? Reaching and *being* in a safe country does not mean *feeling* safe (Cassina and Mochi, 2017). The avalanche does not stop when it meets a small plain, especially if the amount of material is very large. As mentioned earlier, one of the possible consequences of highly critical events or circumstances, such as migration, is that children stop playing, or their possibilities to play with peers are drastically limited. Nonetheless:

> Play gives children the opportunity to change their passivity in the face of events into activity and creativity. In play children can be fully themselves, elaborate and master critical events, have fun, rewrite a reality that they like better and that fits more with their feelings, aspiration and hope.
>
> (Mochi, 2009: 78)

In other words, play is essential to children's recovery, but it cannot happen if children do not feel safe (Panksepp, 1998; Porges, 2011). If children do not feel safe, they are limited in being able to socially engage with others (Porges, 2011) and the longer a child does not feel safe, the situation worsens for a child's psychosocial wellbeing. Therefore, in order to support children, we need first to create a feeling of safety. Creating spaces to play was important since "at each stage of development, it is play and the repeated elements of play that help organize neural systems" (Perry et al., 2000: 10). For the children in our service, some of these necessary experiences were missed along the way, so a supportive process should include as many opportunities to recover them. This consideration and the concept of the enriched environment researched by Diamond (1988) contributed to why the project was extended to all children, parents, and professionals working with them, at multiple levels and to all possible areas of daily life. The approach within the service was broad-based and did not only concern me as the therapeutic play specialist[3] who worked with the most vulnerable families in the centre. An enriched environment has within it, positive relationships, play, and safety which are all macro-elements that can reinforce each other, delineating and contributing to each other (Mochi and Cassina, 2021: 141). An enriched environment can better encourage children's growth, support them in managing difficult situations, and foster their wellbeing allowing their potential to develop.

The project "recovering lost play time": reasons and development

The daily work in the field allowed my colleagues and me to observe hundreds of migrant children over many years. This experience led us to develop a project that was accepted by the board in 2013. We had provided three main reasons to start a five-year project. First, most of the children reaching the centre had significant vulnerabilities and some of them had severe psychological problems that did not decrease over time. Families were constantly exposed to many stressors. As written before, reaching a safe country does not mean feeling safe, nor that all problems are suddenly gone. Our goal was to create the conditions for the avalanche to start slowing down, ultimately to stop, and hopefully to start dissolving.

Second, at that time, there were no interventions inside the centre that could detect promptly and respond effectively to specific children's psychological needs. Moreover, the status of asylum seekers is temporary, which means that by law, an individual can be removed from the country at any time and this status can limit the possibility to access external public services. At the same time, asylum procedures can last several months and this can have a very big impact on the development and wellbeing of a child. Negative experiences in the early years may have permanent consequences (Perry and Pollard, 1997; Perry, 2005), and we wanted to be able to react as soon as possible.

Third, the potential of professionals working with children and families in the centre was not fully utilised. Moreover, the staff felt overwhelmed by critical situations in which they had little chance and capacity of inducing positive change. The group consisted of social workers, teachers, educators, entertainers for children and adolescents, and nurses who were in regular contact with the families and could access information on education, health, social conditions, asylum procedure, and so on. We were used to having daily meetings which provided us with an overall view of each child and family. We knew very little about their past and future, but we were together at that moment and this was a fundamental ingredient to believe in what we could do as professionals and to start putting it into practice.

Before I explain how the project was structured, the kind of activities we implemented, and my story about Samuel (one of the children involved in non-directive play therapy sessions, who recovered his lost play time), I would like to provide underlying reasons for why we started an internal project rather than involving external professionals (apart from the project supervisor and trainers). An internal project overcame the timing issues and the limits imposed by the status of asylum seekers, but it was most of all about the quality and the impact we wanted to achieve through our services to families. Another reason for developing an internal project (rather than involving only external professionals) was the value of the specialised knowledge that experienced professionals acquire in the migration field. I will tell you a brief anecdote to make this point.

> I was asked to organise a meeting with three unaccompanied migrant children aged 15 from Afghanistan. They had been in the centre for five months and I could communicate with them quite easily in Italian (which is the official language in the part of Switzerland the centre is located). I didn't consider it necessary to have an interpreter during the meeting (the topic was not sensitive nor complex) and the boys confirmed that they did not need it. The meeting was held by a board member. He started speaking with them as he usually did in other contexts. I noticed quite soon that the boys could not understand what he was talking about. The board member got particularly nervous when they were not able to answer his questions and he suddenly told me: "Please, translate for them what I'm talking about!". I am skilled in seven languages and Farsi is not one of them, but in fact the boys and I did have a common language. This was possible because I had learned how to communicate with our guests: I choose specific words, modified the rhythm and the tone of my voice, payed attention to their reactions and, if necessary, I repeated my sentences using other words and sometimes by drawing. Maybe you are wondering why I didn't always call an interpreter, since this would seem easier. The answer is that we were doing something more than exchanging information: we were building a relationship, the children were gaining new communication skills or regaining trust in the skills they had. Over time, they could also use them outside the centre and feel able to communicate with others than myself. They had my full attention with no intermediaries, I was able to get to know them better and to adjust my interactions, and they were getting the confirmation to be able to overcome successfully little difficulties, despite everything that has happened to them. They felt active and empowered.

Several authors (Andronico and Guerney, 1969; Brooks and Goldstein, 2015) have highlighted how the relationship that children develop with some educational and supportive figures can have a highly positive impact on their lives. We believed this could happen for the children in our service, if we could acquire new awareness and skills through expanding our knowledge in the psychoeducational field and intentionally using the therapeutic powers of play (Schaefer and Drewes, 2014) to reach specific goals. None of us in the team was a mental health professional (apart from the project supervisor who was a psychologist and registered play therapist supervisor). For those children who were deemed more severe, the training opened up the possibility of using targeted counselling. In fact:

> The specialist in the social, educational, rehabilitative or sanitary field who uses Therapeutic Play in his work adds to his professional prerogatives some

specific methodologies of intervention (extrapolated from the Play Therapy field) with the aim of facilitating the achievement or consolidation of the characteristic objectives of his activity and at the same time offering his clients/interlocutors support in the development of specific skills, mitigating any mild psychological suffering and preventing the development of psychosocial problems.

(Mochi and Cassina, 2021: 149–150)

Step 1

The project was developed by myself (as project manager), in collaboration with the supervisor and the contribution of my colleagues.[4] Step 1 of the project was a needs' assessment. It is indeed very important to have a clear idea of the resources and limitations of the context and the reasons why it would be relevant to start this specific project. I invite the reader to consider the information provided in the previous pages of this chapter: the process of migration, the impact of displacement on families and children, and the need for safety and a safe place to play (see also Chapter 1).

Step 2

In order to start achieving the goals of the project, we planned a series of activities starting the capacity-building process of local child professionals (Mochi and Cassina, 2018). Our role and experience within the centre offered us a privileged position. First, all professionals working with children and parents in the centre followed a training and supervision program tailored to the needs embedded in their professional role. In particular, they were introduced to the relevance of play for children from the neuroscience point of view: how the child's brain develops, why play matters to children, and how to plan developmentally, sensitively, and neurobiologically relevant psychoeducational play-based activities. They became familiar with the concept of the therapeutic powers of play (Schaefer and Drewes, 2014), the levels of intervention for children and parents, and the main play therapy models and tools. Moreover, they were trained in group play therapy (Sweeney et al., 2014) in order to be able to integrate new and appropriate activities and techniques in daily work oriented to specific goals, which were continually monitored and adjusted in response to the group of children. The challenges changed and training included: practice and improve self-regulation and anger management, reduce violent stress reactions, improve communication skills, reduce withdrawal and feelings of fear, improve the ability to understand, elaborate and express feelings, ameliorate problem-solving, and so on.

The professionals were also trained in how to interact with parents, listen to them, and tell them about their children's behaviours and progress and how to deal with daily situations such as limit setting, managing aggressiveness between peers, or dealing with homework for those who were enrolled in school. We tried to be consistent in our attitudes and suggestions and to involve parents as much as possible, even though this was probably one of the most challenging parts of the project. The training program included individual and group supervision. Supervision increased the quality of training as professionals had to transfer what they had learned from the training content to their daily routine working with families. The long-term supervision process has been fundamental to refine the training. It was not enough to learn new amusing play activities and interaction skills, professionals had to know why and when to use the play activities and how to adjust them for a particular group of children to reach specific goals. The intention was to respond to "Paul Gordon's basic question: What treatment, by whom, is the most effective for this individual with this specific problem and in this set of circumstances?" (Drewes, 2021: 7).

Step 3

Shortly after my colleagues started the first module of the training program, we began to modify the environment by creating new play spaces, renovating some existing rooms, and selecting materials. We placed on the desk of the social workers' office a transparent box including mostly sensory materials, miniatures, and white and coloured paper. The box had a magnetic and calming effect on everyone who touched it, even on my own colleagues. We noticed an increase in the number of times people entered the office and the length of time they stayed. The infirmary received new equipment too, especially puppets, dolls, medical kits, and rescue vehicles. The nurses started using play material to interact with children and adolescents during medical checks. We perceived that both children and parents were less scared and more emotionally available before, during, and after the medical procedures and the professionals were able to reach more people and were satisfied with doing their work (D'Antonio, 1984; Webb, 1995).

The teachers provided the classroom with toys. The toys were suited to several areas such as family and care, aggressiveness, creative expression and construction, and multipurpose toys. There were sand trays, miniatures, and water, different kinds of sensory materials (play-doh, clay, fabrics of various textures, colours, and size, and objects from nature such as flowers and dried leaves), materials they considered relevant in children's past and present life, culturally sensitive toys and objects, medical kits, means of transportation, weapons, and human and animal families. Modifying the school environment resulted in making the whole program more efficient. Over time, teachers were also involved in training on how to teach through play. The atmosphere in the classroom was more relaxed and playful and the relationship between teachers and pupils strengthened. The academic results improved and children learnt and practised new skills that were transferred outside the classroom (more information on using therapeutic powers of play in a school context is in Chapter 5).

The centre had a room where educators and entertainers offered weekly play activities for up to 20 children at a time. The space was not particularly big.

In order to limit the possibility of feeling confused or overwhelmed, reduce nonconstructive stimuli, and promote concentration, we decided to reduce the number of toys and materials while diversifying them both culturally and topically. Toys selected facilitated imagination and creativity, were easily accessible, and kept always in the same place. We created a soft corner, which was a little house with pillows and blankets. We split children into groups of a maximum of eight each. The structure of the play activity groups was modified: they started with a ritual at the beginning, something very simple like each child removing shoes, and, later on, a special handshake was inserted for children who wanted to. Then there was a moment of free play with most time being spent in structured activities planned in advance by the professionals according to the age and goals of the group. Depending on how the session proceeded, another moment of free play would be included. The sessions closed with putting the shoes back on and the special handshake. From the second year of the project, we added the time for a little snack. Children took turns carrying snacks and drinks to their peers and returning the glasses to the sink before leaving. This moment turned out to be a great addition, children were involved and felt looked after and empowered.

The educators and entertainers had extra training allowing them to implement structured activities and techniques based on attachment theory where "particular emphasis is placed on positive physical contact as a means of creating connection, involvement, care, regulation, and reassurance" (Mochi and Cassina, 2021: 84). Over time we noticed improvements in both interactions between children and in the quality of their play. In free play, they started interacting more in little groups, they argued less and were less aggressive, played for a longer time, and the play sequences were more complex. During structured activities, they were more focused and involved. The overall atmosphere improved and the need for setting limits decreased. The professionals were more relaxed and playful too.

Play therapy within the service

Modifying the environment included creating a special playroom inside the centre for one-to-one interventions. The room was about 4 metres x 4 metres with basic grey furniture and white empty walls. The room was also used to accommodate emergency cases, which meant our colleagues from the 24/7 surveillance service needed to remove all play materials in a few minutes in order to accommodate new guests. This was limiting, but it pushed us to think and arrange the room strategically. We put a coloured carpet in the middle, we organised different categories of toys in large and small transparent boxes, we placed other toys on a blanket on the bed, and we covered the table with a colourful fabric and arranged large, soft cushions under it. The room was adjusted for each child and according to the play therapy model used.

As the multiple activities continued, the supervision and the regular meetings of the team allowed us to monitor each child and detect those who were considered more vulnerable and needed special attention. We collected all possible information and had a first meeting with parents. As the therapeutic play specialist and head of social services, I was in charge of this part of the process. The first meeting sometimes required the presence of an interpreter. I wanted to be fully respectful of the culture and avoid any misunderstandings. (I take this opportunity to say that, instead, I never invited interpreters inside the playroom, no matter the play therapy model or the age of children. The official language was play.)

I started the meeting by asking parents how they were doing. Some of them were aware that something was wrong and started telling me right away. For others, I asked if they had noticed something unusual. One of my favourite questions to start was: "What does your day in the centre look like so far?". This simple question made them feel calm (it was flexible and everyone could answer it) and gave me hooks to introduce what I wanted to tell them. The next step was to explain our approach and methodologies. I told them about the importance of play for child development and wellbeing and how we could use the therapeutic powers of play to help them overcome difficulties. In the following meeting, I introduced the play therapy model I would use, explained their level of involvement, and together we set the goals. Sometimes the request for help came directly from parents, but unfortunately, this didn't mean that the process started faster or that their availability to be involved was greater.

The professionals' role must be very clear for parents. Collaborating with us in the play therapy process did not increase their chance of acquiring the status of refugee or getting any advantage other than support for their children's wellbeing and hopefully for the whole family. Parents/carers are in a vulnerable position, and we did not want to take advantage of them to get their collaboration. We desire to build a transparent and trusting relationship. Another aspect to keep in mind is that we will never really know what happened in the children's past. I am aware that the more information we have on the clinical history and life experiences of the child and family, the better it is to elaborate a therapeutic plan, but we cannot always rely uniquely on what the family is able or willing to report to us or what is written in the asylum files. For many reasons, the stories do not always match with reality and we could be misguided by inaccurate information. Therefore, we took more time to observe the child in various circumstances and to know the family dynamics. I found it very useful to have family play observations in the special playroom.

Step 4

In the project, parents were involved as much as possible inside and outside the playroom. According to the play therapy methodology applied[5] and parents' availability, they were sometimes my partner in the playroom, other times they were leading the sessions, or they observed only. When the methodology didn't require parents' presence inside the room, I made sure we had regular meetings.

I would be lying if I said it was simple to always get their attention and interest, but I was persistent.

From the second year of the project, educators and entertainers started offering parents the possibility of accompanying them as helpers during walks in the park and day trips in nature with groups of children. Parents were enthusiastic, they felt useful and appreciated and they had fun participating in some of the play activities. The professionals were glad to have motivated helpers and pleasant company. Another activity called "Coffee and tea chats" for (but not limited to) parents, emerged from the parents' involvement. We met once per week to share ideas and experiences on parenthood and children's wellbeing. Most of the participants were women and sometimes they voluntarily prepared sweets for the group. Depending on the topic "chat", I invited my colleagues for coffee too. We always started the meeting with a simple, short, and fun play activity with the aim to break the ice, create a pleasant and relaxed atmosphere, and contribute over time to building a sense of acceptance and belonging to the group. I suggested play activities using miniatures and sand, images, painting supplies, music, and movement. Traditional games guided by the participants were also an appreciated option.

As you can imagine, these four steps are not always chronological, but I hope they gave you the idea of a progression of the activities, starting with the involvement of child professionals and reaching gradually more children and parents. For the last section, I will invite you to the playroom as I describe the story of Samuel, a child I had the privilege to see recovering his lost play time through CCPT.

Case study

In 2014, Samuel was registered as an asylum seeker in Switzerland and transferred with his parents and his newborn sister to the centre I was working in. The family situation was complex and fraught, shaped and consolidated during a long and unpredictable migratory process. Parents were anxious, stressed, frustrated by the whole situation, physically and mentally tired, and violent with each other. The surveillance service of the centre intervened weekly in the night to quell the fights between them. The family lived in a room with a small kitchen in the corner, two beds, a closet, a table, four chairs, and a balcony. The days did not have regular rhythms; the meals were not cooked nor consumed together. The child opened the refrigerator when he felt hungry and ate wherever he happened to be and often on the floor. The bedtimes were random; Samuel stayed up very often until late and fell asleep at different times during the day. Neither mother nor father took care of his hygiene. The father started a temporary job quite soon after their arrival, and the mother was focused on the newborn.

Samuel was highly neglected. He looked fearful, withdrawn, and stressed. He was very aggressive with his peers during group activities and with his sister too. He always had a serious and constricted facial expression and severe evacuation difficulties. He showed understanding of his native and local language, but, despite being three years old, he had never uttered a single word. The paediatric examination detected a slight delay in physical development and what they called "a difficulty of an unspecified nature related to language". One morning, his mother walked into my office and asked me: "Why doesn't he talk?". I realised that this was the ideal moment to suggest a play therapy intervention to the family. I didn't know if the parents were ready for it (who can ever be "ready" for it?), how much they would be available and for how long, and I could not confirm that the child would start talking, but they were concerned and I had their attention.

In order to prepare myself, to have a clear overview of the process, and to be able to facilitate, guide, and involve the parents, I used a chart (see Table 3.1 as an example). I had developed this table for a project in 2013 and had applied it on many other occasions, including teaching master students. I will share it briefly with you since I believe it can be useful. The structure of it is very simple: the first column is named "Observations". Here we insert any relevant information we collect that can give us a clear idea about the child and family conditions, resources, and limits. The second column called "Goals", is about the opportunities for improvement from the observations made. We fill it with the goals set for the child and parents. The third column is dedicated to the "Indicators". This involves verifying the goals defined through observations inside and outside the playroom. This step is fundamental to monitor the play therapy process and to adjust if necessary. It is also to guide the parents in what to observe, how to be involved, and to keep them motivated by becoming able to notice small changes. The fourth column is called "Other" and can

Table 3.1 Recovering lost play time chart (or "RLPT chart").

Observations	Goals	Indicators	Other
The child is 3 years old and does not communicate verbally. He shows a good understanding of both original language and Italian.	Expand and reinforce non-verbal communication skills and acquire verbal communication skills.	Did the child start doing anything different from before? Did he develop new strategies to communicate? If yes, are they the same with you (parents), his sister, and his peers? If he started making noises or using words: which ones, with who, and on what occasion? How does he (and you) react to them? Did he widen his vocabulary? How many words does he use now? Is he using sentences and when?	The father started a new job and now the child spends most of the day with his mother and sister.

include any relevant information such as some important changes or events in family life.

The assessment of circumstances, needs, and resources suggested CCPT as being the more suitable methodology. CCPT is a non-directive methodology that assumes that in a safe and accepting environment, children will grow in the direction of health. The professional (therapist) creates a relationship-oriented climate showing genuineness, acceptance, and unconditional positive regard and trust that children can solve their own problems (VanFleet et al., 2010). We agreed on two weekly 30-minute sessions in the special playroom until the goals, which were set together with the parents, were accomplished. The goals were as follows:

- Feel accepted and gain a feeling of safety.
- Perceive and practice control over the context.
- Improve self-esteem and self-confidence.
- Ameliorate the ability to express and manage feelings such as stress and frustration.
- Develop non-verbal communication skills.
- Acquire verbal communication skills.
- Have the possibility to relax and amuse.

My agenda included objectives for the parents too (which I noted in the column "Goals"). They were not fully aware of their child's needs, especially that of feeling safe, and I wanted them to feel more competent and helpful in resolving their son's issues. We started by building a daily routine: cook one meal a day and eat it all together at the table; buy a toothbrush and accompany Samuel while brushing his teeth every day before going to bed; prepare a box of toys for his exclusive use and keep it always in the same corner of the room. In our second meeting, I explained that having rhythms and positive routines foster predictability and this is an essential component for making children feel safe. If their son felt safer (meaning less focus on unpredictable and fearful risk factors), he would be able to play more, and to learn new fundamental skills through play and, hopefully, to start speaking. I explained simply how a child's brain worked, to help increase the comprehension of a couple of scared parents who were themselves living in highly critical circumstances.

The first eight minutes of the first session Samuel was standing still at the entry of the room, looking repeatedly at me and the toys, and wringing his hands. I was sitting quietly close to him while doing empathic listening: "You don't know what to do", "You are curious", "There are many toys and you like them", and "You are wondering what you can do here". I did not want to rescue him in this difficult moment by giving a solution. I wanted instead to convey that I accepted the way he felt, that it was all right to feel uncertain and not knowing what to do. At the eighth minute, I moved my head in the direction of the toys and looked around in silence. Samuel started slowly taking steps towards the centre of the room, I followed him. During the session, he would continuously pick up toys, bring them to me without making any noise, play action or request, and put them back exactly where he found them. He seemed curious but very insecure, and he needed always to look at me. To make him feel safer, I had to maintain my congruence in the way I was using empathic listening and remain mindful of all those non-verbal signals (posture, mimic, tone, and rhythm of voice) that could communicate that I felt calm and regulated with my social engagement system activated (Porges, 2011; Kestly, 2014). I had to keep in mind that as a professional, we can act as "safer bank" for our clients (Mochi, forthcoming 2022).

In the second and third sessions, Samuel reached the centre of the room without hesitation, but a similar pattern followed. I sensed he felt more secure with me. I didn't know if he wasn't able to play with the play materials or if he didn't feel safe enough to do so yet. In the fourth session, the first significant change occurred as he involved me in a play action: he pulled a toy cream dispenser closer to me and pressed with his finger to let me know he wanted me to put cream on. I started spreading the cream on my hands and then on my arms. He seemed amused and moved the dispenser closer to my face, so I put the cream there too. Then he turned to the kitchen corner, grabbed a spoon and a plate, put a toy chicken leg on it, and brought it closer to my mouth. I accepted the invitation and pretended to eat. I must admit that I felt relieved, he knew how to use pretend play abilities and how to request my involvement. Looking at the "indicators" column, I perceived the process was moving along.

From the sixth session, Samuel left most of the toys where he played. He even tried to purposefully break some of them while looking at me and waiting for my reaction. He began to show interest in new toys such as the phone, a rabbit mask, paper and paints, and the gun, but the main theme of the sessions was still care and nurture. He was a different child, eager to touch and experiment by playing. His play was mostly typical of younger children, he was focused on sensory-motor activities as he built an understanding of the objects around him and their functions (Stagnitti, 2021).

Starting from the ninth session, Samuel began to make exclamations and pronounce short words including: "here, this, that, hey, up". More than anything, in this session, the play and theme changed: the child shot me repeatedly with the gun. I fell to the floor, and every time I tried to say something or even to move, he would shoot me again. I lay on the floor for most of the time, then he suddenly took a box and came to me saying: "Hey, up, up" tapping his hand on my head to get me up. He handed me the box letting me know with a gesture that he wanted me to open it. I made attempts saying it wasn't easy and he suggested I do it with my teeth. I still couldn't do it, and he snorted by folding his arms on his chest in disapproval. I told him: "You are really annoyed that I cannot open this box". When we finally managed to open it he exclaimed with satisfaction: "Oh, wow!". In CCPT, "play themes are patterns or instances of a child's play that appear to have meaning for the child" (VanFleet et al., 2010: 88), and it seemed to me that from this session, Samuel could finally experience the feeling of being powerful and in control of the situation.

After about ten sessions, the parents and my colleagues started reporting improvements in different areas: the child was less aggressive with his peers and sister, he appeared more serene and smiling, and he was more regular in evacuation. One day, the father run into my office and screamed: "Samuel called me dad!". Developments in the playroom were beginning to have visible effects on the outside, and this was very well perceived by everyone involved. It especially gave his parents motivation to keep on doing little adjustments in the family daily routine.

At the thirteenth session, Samuel hit me with a rubber sword, shot the snake with the gun, stroked the tiger, and then pretended to be afraid of it and hid behind me. At the end of the session, he insisted angrily to stay in the playroom, and although he struggled a lot to put his own shoes on, he refused to be helped and said: "Leave, they're mine!". In the following sessions, he showed increasingly complex play with logical sequences. In the eighteenth session, the play theme changed again. He put the bib on *Ken*, he stroked it and said: "It's my dad". He asked me to put a bib on him too, and after that, he sat on my legs and let go. I gently hugged him and began to rock him. When he was quiet with his eyes closed, I could not help thinking how much he was in need of regaining those missed developmental experiences (Perry and Hambrick, 2008), and especially feeling cared for and loved. After a couple of minutes, he moved and I immediately spread my arms. He looked at me and went and got more toys. He spent most of the session lying on my lap. In the last few minutes, he sang a song using the megaphone, then gave it to me letting me know that it was my turn. I sang an improvised, wordless melody like his. He looked at me smiling, and when I finished he said, "There!" and took the megaphone back.

I didn't imagine that was our last session, the process was not complete. After a first exploratory phase, Samuel completed an aggressive phase and was currently exploring the regressive one. He still hadn't reached what Louise Guerney (1983) called the "mastery phase". A couple of days after the eighteenth session, Samuel was urgently hospitalised due to a domestic accident. After recovering, the authority removed him and his sister from their parents and from the centre. The play therapy process was interrupted as well as any other form of contact. After a couple of months, the country decided that the whole family must be expelled from Switzerland because the asylum request was not accepted.

Three years after their departure, I was having a meeting in a colleague's office. On my way out, I saw a child of about 6 years old. He looked at me and said: "Hi". Samuel was back in Switzerland with his mother, father, and sister. He had grown a lot. He was slender, he looked me in the eye, and he seemed embarrassed but determined. After this first unexpected meeting, I saw Samuel again for some months before the family was expelled from Switzerland again. I heard him talking and telling funny stories; I saw him playing happily with peers and interacting quietly with his sister. One day we were sitting next to each other on the stairs in the courtyard, he looked at me and asked: "Is it true that you and I played together when I was little? My mum told me. Was I good at playing?". I smiled at him and replied: "I remember very well when we used to play together. You did a lot of different games and you knew exactly what to do. I really enjoyed playing with you".

Considerations and limits of the project

The end of the chapter is approaching and with that, I would like to share some considerations and limits of such a project and approach. One first consideration is that every adaptation and structural change needs time, the more time you have the better. Starting such a project means a co-constructed process of deconstruction and reconstruction. In Chapter 1, this process is discussed in more depth and this is why I will not cover this here, except to say that the exceptional dynamism of the migration field needs to be underlined. The huge number of individuals' and families' needs and the limited time available can have an impact, especially on the willingness of institutions to commit to this kind of project. The type of centre I worked in is the ideal place to start a play intervention because there are key human resources and it is the first step for families after their registration in a new country. We know how important it is, especially for children, to benefit from responsive and early interventions.

At the same time, it is temporary accommodation. Families are there while waiting for an answer to the asylum request which can be positive or negative. In either case, they will have to leave the centre. Is it worthwhile to implement a project for families who will not stay long? Is it the right moment for parents to be involved in such a process considering the complexity of their lives and everything they are still worried about? Moreover, how difficult and frustrating is it for the professionals to be involved with children and parents at such a deep level knowing they could be removed at any time and gone for good? I have my answers after meeting Samuel again. Seeing him again, I could see that the project made perfect sense, that it is always worthwhile to plant a seed, no matter how the ground appears.

But is this enough for every player involved in the complex world of migration? The structure of the project was well conceived and well executed. The results with children and families were extraordinary. In retrospect, I see that something was missing. When I resigned to devote myself fully to the world of play therapy, nobody took my leadership position. The training of new professionals in play therapy methodologies was not embedded within the service to address needs and interests when a new influx of unaccompanied migrant children aged 13–17 came to Europe. New migrant families continue to arrive, and I can only hope that, mindful of the past, the organisation will be willing to integrate the therapeutic powers of play as a common language and a foundation for a new professional culture.

Conclusion

The migration process, as well as other kinds of crises, is sometimes so complex and enduring that it becomes the only life children know. Difficult situations and prolonged stress can cause permanent structural changes in children's psyche and brain morphology, affecting them at emotional and behavioural levels and limiting their possibilities of wellbeing. Nevertheless, although we cannot change the past and affect the outcome of the asylum procedure (what is referred to as the "nature of the situation" in Chapter 1), we can trigger a positive change in families' lives by working on individual factors inside the playroom and factors in the support system outside the playroom. The project described is an example of how applying the therapeutic powers of play and play therapy interventions can result in a chain of positive outcomes and its principles can be applied to other kinds of critical contexts.

"Recovering lost play time" is not only based on the importance of widening the possibilities for children in vulnerable situations to benefit from the power of play. It also includes the assumption that child professionals develop new skills to benefit families as a whole because of highly effective interactions and assessment of their emotional and developmental needs and, when necessary, from individual play therapy interventions in the special playroom. In this way, children are given a better chance of recovering and developing their potential and parents a greater sense of safety, awareness, and satisfaction in their valuable role.

Notes

1 The status of "asylum seeker" and "refugee" are two distinct moments of the same procedure. An asylum seeker is "an individual who is seeking international protection. In countries with individualized procedures, an asylum seeker is someone whose claim has not yet been finally decided on by the country in which he or she has submitted it. Not every asylum seeker will ultimately be recognized as a refugee, but every recognized refugee is initially an asylum seeker" (IOM, 2021).
2 Neither the author of this chapter or its contents are politically oriented. The experiences presented aim to underline the potential of the therapeutic powers of play and play therapy in a highly vulnerable context such us forced migration and forced displacement. The assumptions and the intervention presented can be applied to similar complex psychosocial conditions.
3 A "Therapeutic Play Specialist" (TP-S) is a professional with a degree in social, educational, rehabilitative, or health field trained and supervised in play therapy methodologies that have gone through an accreditation process recognised by one or more national associations' members of the International Consortium of Play Therapy Associations (IC-PTA).
4 The information in this section has been extrapolated from the internal reports avoiding all personal references, organised and completed by the author of this chapter.
5 The play therapy methodologies applied were Child-Centered Play Therapy (VanFleet et al., 2010), Filial Therapy (VanFleet and Guerney, 2003), and Learn to Play Therapy (Stagnitti, 2021). Sandtray Therapy (Homeyer and Sweeney, 2016) and Theraplay® (Booth and Jernberg, 2010) activities and techniques were applied in other areas of the project.

References

Andronico, M.P. and Guerney, B.G. (1969) 'The potential application of filial therapy to the school situation', in B.G., Guerney (ed.) *Psychotherapeutic agents: New roles for nonprofessionals, parents and teachers*, New York, NY: Holt, Rinehart & Winston, 371–377.

Booth, P.B. and Jernberg, A.M. (2010) *Theraplay: Helping parents and children build better relationships through attachment-based play*, 3rd edn., San Francisco, CA: John Wiley & Sons, Inc.

Brooks, R. and Goldstein, S. (2015) 'The power of mindsets. Guideposts for a resilience-based treatment approach', in D.A., Crenshaw, R., Brooks and S., Goldstein (eds.) *Play therapy interventions to enhance resilience*, New York, NY: The Guilford Press, 168–193.

Brown, S. and Vaughan, C. (2009) *Play: How it shapes the brain, opens the imagination, and invigorates the soul*, New York, NY: Penguin.

Cassina, I. (2015) *Due parole con lo psicologo* [online audio directory], available: www.spreaker.com/user/radiobullets/due-parole-con-lo-psicologo-5-rubrica [accessed 3 November 2021].

Cassina, I. (2019) 'Bambini migranti: Recuperare il tempo di gioco perduto', training presented for the *Master in Play Therapy*, INA International Academy for Play Therapy studies and Psychosocial Projects, Rome, 23–24 March 2019.

Cassina, I. and Mochi, C. (2017) *The use of play therapy with migrant children in centres for asylum seekers in Switzerland*, conference, Brampton, Canada, 25 October 2017.

D'Antonio, I. (1984) 'Therapeutic use of play in hospitals', *Nursing clinics of North America*, 19, 351–359.

Diamond, M.C. (1988) *Enriching heredity: The impact of the environment on the anatomy of the brain*, New York, NY: Free Press.

Drewes, A. (2021) 'Therapeutic powers of play', *Rivista di Play Therapy*, 2, May 2021, 7–12.

Encyclopædia Britannica, Inc. (2021) *Avalanche*, available: www.britannica.com/science/avalanche [accessed 3 September 2021].

Erikson, E.H. (1950) *Childhood and society*, New York, NY: Norton.

Goleman, D. (1997) *The emotional intelligence*, New York, NY: Bantam books.

Guerney, L.F. (1983) 'Child-centered (non directive) play therapy', in C.E., Schaefer and K.J., O'Connor (eds.) *Handbook of play therapy*, 1, New York, NY: John Wiley & Sons, 21–64.

Homeyer, L.E. and Sweeney, D.S. (2016) *Sandtray therapy: A practical manual*, 3rd edn., New York, NY: Routledge.

International Organization for Migration IOM (2021) *Key migration terms*, available: www.iom.int/key-migration-terms [accessed 2 September 2021].

Kestly, T. (2014) *The interpersonal neurobiology of play: Brain-building interventions for emotional well-being*, New York, NY: Norton.

Landreth, G.L. (2002) *Play therapy: The art of the relationship*, 2nd edn., Philadelphia, PA: Brunner/Routledge.

Mochi, C. (2009) 'Trauma repetition: Intervention in psychological safe places', *Eastern Journal of Psychiatry*, 12(1&2), 75–80.

Mochi, C. (forthcoming 2022) *Beyond the clouds: An autoethnographic research exploring the good practice in crisis settings*, Ann Arbor, MI: Loving Healing Press.

Mochi, C. and Cassina, I. (2018) *Play therapy around the globe: International crisis work with children*, training presented at Northwest Center for Play Therapy Studies Summer Institute, George Fox University, Portland, 6 June 2018.

Mochi, C. and Cassina, I. (2021) *Introduzione alla play therapy. Quando il gioco è la terapia*, Lugano: INA Play Therapy Press.

Panksepp, J. (1998) *Affective neuroscience: The foundations of human and animal emotions*, New York, NY: Oxford University.

Perry, B.D. (2005) 'Maltreatment and the developing child: How early childhood experience shapes child and culture', *Centre for Children and Families in the Justice system*, 1–6.

Perry, B.D. and Hambrick, E.P. (2008) 'The neurosequential model of therapeutics', *Reclaiming Children and Youth*, 17(3), 38–43.

Perry, B.D., Hogan, L. and Marlin, S. (2000) 'Curiosity, pleasure and play: A neurodevelopmental perspective', *Haaeyc Advocate*, 20, 9–12.

Perry, B.D. and Pollard, R.A. (1997) 'Altered brain development following global neglect in early childhood', *Society for Neuroscience*, Proceedings from Annual Meeting, New Orleans.

Porges, S. (2011) *The polyvagal theory: Neurophysiological foundations of emotions, attachment, communication, and self-regulation*, New York, NY: Norton.

Schaefer, C.E. and Drewes, A.A. (eds.) (2014) *The therapeutic powers of play: 20 core agents of change*, Hoboken, NJ: John Wiley and Sons.

Stagnitti, K. (2021) *Learn to play therapy: Principles, process and practical activities*, 2nd edn., Melbourne: Learn to Play.

Sweeney, D.S., Baggerly, J. and Ray, D.C. (2014) *Group play therapy: A dynamic approach*, New York, NY: Routledge.

VanFleet, R. and Guerney, L. (2003) *Casebook of filial therapy*, Boiling Springs, PA: Play Therapy Press.

VanFleet, R., Sywulak, A.E. and Sniscak, C.C. (eds.) (2010) *Child-centered play therapy*, New York, NY: The Guilford Press.

Webb, J.R. (1995) 'Play therapy with hospitalized children', *International Journal of Play Therapy*, 4(1), 51–59.

Webb, N.B. (2007) 'The family and community context of children facing crisis or trauma', in N.B., Webb (ed.) *Play therapy with children in crisis: Individual, group, and family treatment*, New York, NY: The Guilford Press, 3–20.

4 Tele-Play Therapy

Principles of remote interventions using the therapeutic powers of play

Kate L. Renshaw and Judi A. Parson

In Section 1, the principles for remote Tele-Play Therapy are established. First, play therapists should initially familiarise themselves with the scaffolded approach to telecommunications for play therapy. The second step is reviewing the guiding principles which set out both practice guidelines and contraindications for using telecommunications in play therapy. The third is to consider and prepare the three Tele-Play Therapy practice environments, namely, the practitioner, the child client, and the virtual setting. Finally, a diverse range of telecommunication practice considerations is given. To highlight these principles in action, a composite case example is offered in Section 2. Henry is the focal point of this remote Tele-Play Therapy intervention; the therapeutic powers of play are aligned with his biopsychosocial health needs within the context of his family.

In 2019, the authors contributed to a chapter on the use of technology in play therapy. At that time, we stated that "the world of multi-media and technology has knocked on the therapeutic practitioner's consulting room door" (Parson et al., 2019: 64). With the onset of the Covid-19 global pandemic in 2020, the virtual world and digital methods have irrevocably transformed: (1) the avenues to access play therapy; (2) the appearance of the door to the playroom; and (3) the boundaries of play therapy. The already dynamic nature of the world increased in intensity overnight, which altered both opportunities and challenges in activating the therapeutic powers of play (TPoP) and, therefore, necessitated the need for clear principles for Tele-Play Therapy practice (Schaefer and Drewes, 2014).

It is hard to imagine what the reaction might have been to Tele-Play Therapy from some of the scholars who informed the development of play therapy, such as Virginia Axline (1969) and Clark Moustakas (1959). Could they have even conceived that the playroom would one-day transition into the virtual environment? Or was this virtual environment perhaps more akin to the science fiction writings of H.G. Wells? Coincidentally, over 100 years ago, this famous futuristic writer also published a key text *Floor Games* (Wells, 1911), which influenced Margaret Lowenfeld, a paediatrician and pioneer of child psychotherapy and play therapy. Inspired by the writings of H.G. Wells, Lowenfeld created the World Technique, known in play therapy as sandplay/sand tray and more recently in digitised forms such as the Virtual Sandtray App (VSA) and

DOI: 10.4324/9781003252375-5

the online Sand Tray, both of which are detailed further in the Applications (Apps) section of this chapter (Hutton, 2004; Turner, 2004).

There is no doubt that play therapy in a playroom and Tele-Play Therapy in a virtual space are two vastly different approaches to therapeutic interventions. However, the strong philosophical similarities between play therapy practice in a physical playroom and Tele-Play Therapy practice using telecommunications ground the therapist within the context of their modality. They are both based on the premise that therapists meet their clients where they are presently located developmentally and emotionally. Telecommunications in play therapy broadens the geographical reach of play therapy practice through the digital landscape. For this reason, principles are vital to guide and distinguish between the physicality of play therapy to the digitisation of Tele-Play Therapy.

Amid this change, humanistic play therapy skills (HPTS) and the TPoP have remained an anchor point tethering the physical and virtual realms of this newly expanded play therapy universe (Axline, 1964, 1969; Rogers, 1957; Moustakas, 1959; Winnicott, 1965, 1971; Schaefer and Drewes, 2014). As described by Renshaw and Parson (2021: 76), "Humanistic Play Therapy Skills and the Therapeutic Powers of Play complement each other to form the art and science of Play Therapy". As a reference point for this chapter, the 20 TPoPs (Schaefer and Drewes, 2014) are categorised under four domains, namely, facilitates communication, increases personal strengths, fosters emotional wellness, and enhances social relationships. The therapeutic powers of play (see Figure 4.1) schemata is a useful quick reference for the 20 TPoPs under the four domains. A publicly available short video presentation can be accessed on YouTube-https://youtube.com/watch?v=wuu59E97igU&feature=share

Historical evolution of Tele-Play Therapy

In the mid-20th century, human society transitioned from the industrial age to the information age, also known as the digital age. By the 1990s, E-health defined the use of information technology in healthcare practice (Barak et al., 2008). E-health encompasses Tele-Health, Tele-medicine, Tele-psychology, e-therapy, and many more digital health services (Maeder and Smith, 2010). M-health refers to the inclusion of mobile technologies into healthcare including mobile phones, text messaging, e-mails, and so on. An ever-expanding array of information technologies facilitate the delivery of E-health and M-health services (Field, 1996). Information technologies typically fall into two categories, i.e. hardware or software. Hardware includes telephones/mobile phones, computers/laptops, tablets, headsets/earphones, pen/stylus, cameras, microphone, mouse, keyboard, game controllers, printer/scanner, and so on. Software is operating systems such as apps, programs, search engines, electronic storage facilities, and so on. Common E-health and M-health communication methods such as text messaging, e-mail, and video conferencing rely on both hardware and software technologies.

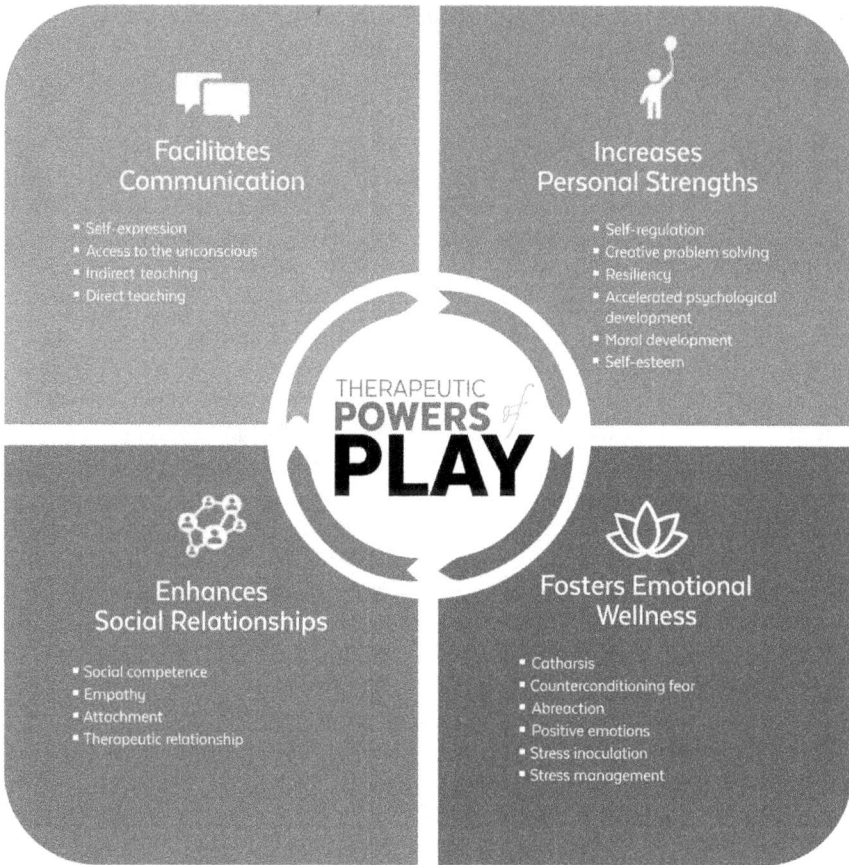

Figure within the image:

Facilitates Communication
- Self-expression
- Access to the unconscious
- Indirect teaching
- Direct teaching

Increases Personal Strengths
- Self-regulation
- Creative problem solving
- Resiliency
- Accelerated psychological development
- Moral development
- Self-esteem

THERAPEUTIC POWERS of PLAY

Enhances Social Relationships
- Social competence
- Empathy
- Attachment
- Therapeutic relationship

Fosters Emotional Wellness
- Catharsis
- Counterconditioning fear
- Abreaction
- Positive emotions
- Stress inoculation
- Stress management

© Parson, Renshaw & Zimmer (2020)

Figure 4.1 The therapeutic powers of play.

Source: Infographic created by Parson et al. (2020a). An earlier version is Parson, J. (2017) 'Puppet play therapy: Integrating Theory, Evidence and Action (ITEA)', presented at the International Play Therapy Study Group, Champneys at Forest Mere, England. June 18, Adapted from Schaefer, C.E. and Drewes, A.A. (2014) *The therapeutic powers of play: 20 core agents of change*, 2nd edn., Hoboken, NJ: Wiley.

Section 1: principles of Tele-Play Therapy

Prior to the Covid-19 global pandemic, a significant population served by E-health and M-health were identified as geographically remote communities. Between 2010 and 2020, the field of play therapy was starting to make some initial moves into the E-health arena; some clinicians were already offering Tele-Health services, utilising text messaging or email, engaging in online video conference clinical supervision, accessing virtual professional development, and engaging in play therapy blended training programs which included online delivery of teaching materials (Parson and Hickson, 2016; Glazer, 2017; Stone, 2019, 2020, 2021).

In 2015, the authors co-presented therapeutic text messaging in play therapy at the Australasia Pacific Play Therapy Association (APPTA) Conference (Renshaw et al., 2015). During this presentation, the audience was invited to participate in a paper-based questionnaire survey. Of the 20 respondents (n = 20), 17 (85%) identified as play therapists. The respondents provided their views on therapeutic texting; however, some survey information was extracted on Tele-Play Therapy. Just over half of the respondents had used texting; in order of frequency, the most common reasons for texting use were appointment reminders, relationship enhancement, and engagement to attend sessions. Three-quarters of respondents did not allow mobile phones into the playroom during play therapy sessions. Common uses of mobile phones or tablets in play therapy were to facilitate the inclusion of music, photography, or digital art making in sessions. The main concerns cited by respondents regarding the inclusion of therapeutic texting or other information technologies as part of play therapy sessions were focused on boundary and confidentiality issues. Other concerns raised by respondents included the age of their child clients, the technological preferences of the parents, the possible distraction of technology, and the potential legalities. Three respondents noted that this was new terrain for them, but they were curious and open to incorporating information technologies into clinical practice. Suggestions by the respondents for developing information technologies in play therapy included the need for clear contracting and organisational policies; clear professional policies and guidelines provided by registration bodies, informed by relevant laws; professional development training in digital play therapy practice; guidance on maintenance of professional boundaries in the digital space; and a live/updatable repository of suitable digital resources. This survey was conducted 2015, and it would be interesting to conduct another questionnaire to assess changing opinions in this short timeframe, indicating the rapidly changing world and dynamic environment we work in.

During the Covid-19 global pandemic, which commenced in early 2020, knowledge was rapidly transferred from E-health and M-health into as many health services as feasible for continuous health care throughout periods of lockdowns and restrictions. Many of the pre-pandemic concerns highlighted by clinicians, organisations, professional registration or licencing bodies, and even governments around digital health practices quickly eroded. A rapid change occurred in policy that guided practice, industry standards, and the accessibility of digital hardware and software to facilitate service delivery. In response to the pandemic, registration bodies provided practice guidance to support clinicians to adapt to the changing digital landscape. One example is the Australasia Pacific Play Therapy Association's (APPTA's) COVID-19 (Coronavirus) – APPTA Advice to Members (Renshaw and Parson, 2020). In March 2020, the authors of this publication advised that Tele-Play Therapy was in a phase of rapid development in response to the pandemic conditions (Ibid.). They proposed the following working definition:

> Tele-Play Therapy is telecommunications for Play Therapists . . . Emerging electronic communication networked technology, which requires audiovisual functionality, enables Play Therapists to engage in a range of telecommunications at the appropriate scaffolded level: 1) Tele-Play; 2) Tele-Health; and 3) Tele-Play Therapy. The use of reliable hardware and encrypted software is paramount in the provision of this service.
>
> (Renshaw and Parson, 2020: para. 2)

We propose the addition of a fourth level, 4) Tele-Filial Therapy, be added to this definition.

As the Covid-19 global pandemic intensified, it was recommended that APPTA members "consider their individual scope of practice and base any therapeutic decisions on public health guidance, Tele-Health recommendations and the current research on disaster service delivery" (Renshaw and Parson, 2020: para. 2). We can draw on the knowledge generated during the pandemic to inform future remote play therapy interventions. Table 4.1 extends on the "Reflexivity when considering Play Therapy roles during an ongoing crisis" table and has been adapted for the purpose of this chapter (Van-Fleet and Mochi, 2015; Renshaw and Parson, 2020: para. 3). Reflecting on the considerations for remote Tele-Play Therapy interventions supports clinicians to ensure practice occurs within their scope of practice. These considerations could potentially uncover important clinical aspects to examine, adapt, or extend their scope of practice through knowledge acquisition, technical skills, and practical experience.

Telecommunications for play therapy

The three scaffolded levels of the APPTA telecommunications for play therapy definition plus the newly included fourth level are now outlined in further detail, namely: 1) Tele-Play; 2) Tele-Health; 3) Tele-Play Therapy; and 4) Tele-Filial Therapy. Careful assessment is needed to ascertain the appropriate Tele-Play Therapy intervention for each child and family system. Contraindicators at each scaffolded level should be assessed and fully considered.

Tele-Play

"Play Therapists understand play. Of any group of psychologically focused professionals, Play Therapists know more about the intricacies, nuances, fundamentals, and processes of play than anyone else" (Stone, 2020: 1). For this reason, play therapists are ideally suited to provide Tele-Play interventions. However, there is currently confusion with terms such as Tele-Play and

Table 4.1 Considerations for remote Tele-Play Therapy interventions.

Remote Tele-Play Therapy interventions	Consideration
Identify local services that can also support this intervention.	Can the remote play therapy intervention complement local service provision?
Align with government legislation, policies, and practice recommendations for the country, state, or territory.	Does the scope of practice need to be considered and practice adjusted?
Tele-Play	What playful recreational activities or guidance can support families?
Assess	Which assessments are needed to gauge suitability for remote interventions?
Assist in planning and delivery of playful activities.	How can the play therapist support families and/ or communities to provide playful interactions?
Offer consultation and advice for selecting creative play resources that will meet the needs of children, families, and communities.	Which developmentally and culturally sensitive toys and play resources are useful to align with suggested playful activities?
Access clinical supervision and professional development training with consideration to their intended scope of practice.	What are your areas of expertise? What do you need to consider within clinical supervision in preparation for remote interventions? What additional professional development is needed?
When assessed as appropriate, deliver the selected remote interventions for children, families, and/or the community.	How will you deliver the selected remote intervention? What planning is needed for the child/children, family, and community?

Tele-Play Therapy being used interchangeably. Mullen (2021: 253) offers one definition:

> Tele-Play Therapy refers to the use of a systematic approach to Play Therapy using play and Play Therapy interventions in a virtual context by a professional mental health practitioner expressly trained in Play Therapy. Teleplay would refer to use of the systematic approaches to Play Therapy and use of Play Therapy interventions, the difference in Teleplay is that the clinician has not been specifically trained in play therapy.

However, for the purpose of this chapter, we are proposing that when used in a systematic and scaffolded way, Tele-Play can be part of a play therapist's tele-communications repertoire. We offer the following definition:

> Tele-Play delivered by a Play Therapist is a carefully selected format of play using telecommunications with the goal of facilitating a playful, relational connection with the child whilst supporting the family within the context of their unique family structure.

The Play Therapy Hourglass schemata (see Figure 4.2) is a useful tool when defining Tele-Play and differentiating it from Tele-Play Therapy. The hourglass provides a visual distinction between play therapy in the top half of the hourglass and therapeutic, educative, and normative play in the lower half of the hourglass. The downward arrow on the right-hand side indicates the professional application of play therapy in other domains of play. The hourglass can be used by play therapists to consider the scope of practice as well as guide the planning and sequencing of Tele-Play interventions.

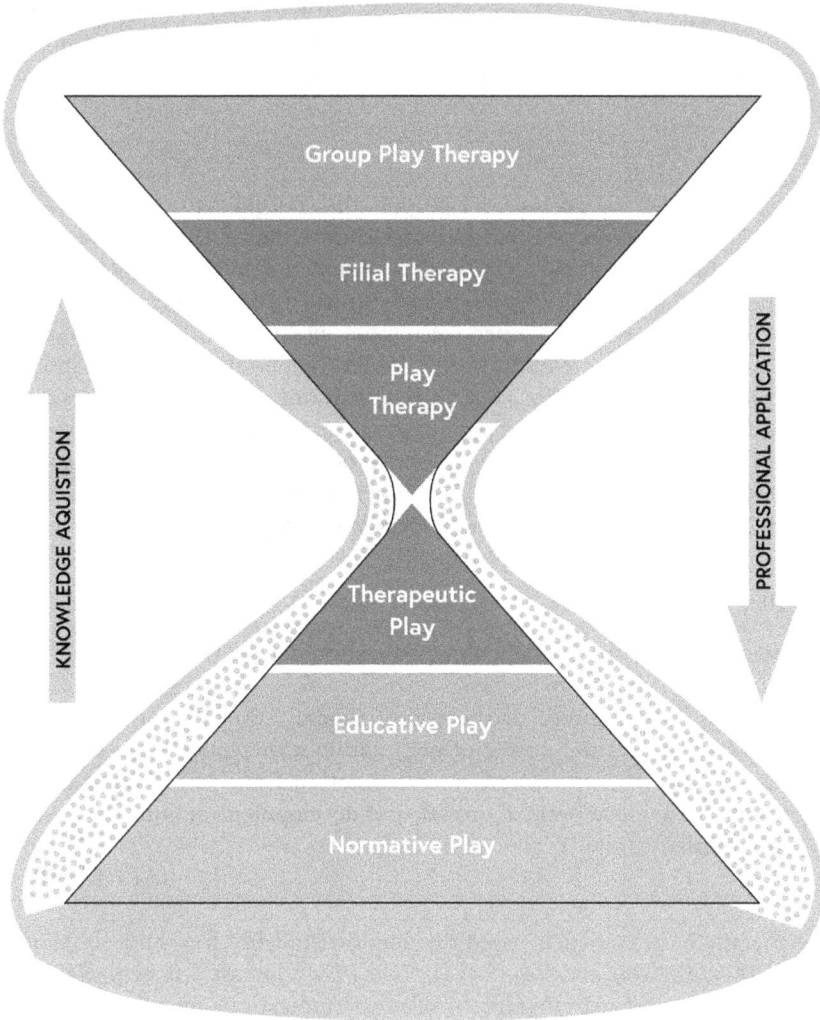

Figure 4.2 Play Therapy Hourglass.

Source: Graphic created by Parson et al. (2018).

Tele-Play interventions may consist of the play therapist "being with" a child for a structured amount of time and consist of playful activities or games. Humanistic play therapy skills are still used during a Tele-Play intervention. Prior to the Tele-Play intervention, planning should occur between the play therapist and the child's caregivers. Consider an appropriate physical space for the Tele-Play sessions and where other members of the household will be at the time (including the whereabouts of household pets). Discuss hardware, software, and teleconferencing platform options. Ensure a trial of telecommunications occurs prior to the first Tele-Play session. An emergency contact phone number that can be used during Tele-Play sessions is essential should the play therapist need to contact the caregivers. Discuss and explore what art, craft, and play resources are suitable (making sure to discuss the potential for mess with certain expressive materials).

Tele-Health

In remote play therapy practice, we propose that Tele-Health refers to both the delivery and facilitation of healthcare service provision using telecommunications. Tele-Health sessions are typically conducted between the play therapist and the child's caregivers, which is referred to as the therapeutic alliance. Supporting caregivers is a vital aspect of remote interventions (Mochi and VanFleet, 2009). Thus, we recommend Tele-Health appointments be included in both Tele-Play and Tele-Play Therapy interventions. A range of services can be provided during Tele-Health appointments; examples include intake meetings, administration of assessments, therapeutic progress meetings (reviewing therapeutic work to date and offering recommendations), parent support sessions, psychoeducation sessions, and final discharge meetings.

Tele-Play Therapy

The Australasia Pacific Play Therapy Association defines play therapy as

> founded on a number of theoretical models whereby the trained Play Therapist utilises the power of play, within a therapeutic relationship, to relieve suffering, prevent or resolve emotional and behavioural difficulties and to achieve optimal growth and development of children (or older individuals).
>
> (APPTA, 2014a)

Play therapy is an evidence-based therapeutic modality for children (Bratton et al., 2005; Bratton and Lin, 2015). Tele-Play Therapy has been described as a virtual form of play therapy or telecommunications for play therapy. As Tele-Play Therapy is an emerging therapeutic approach, efficacy and comparability to traditional play therapy practice methods are at this stage only hypothesised.

Stone (2021: xiv) proposed collapsing the multitude of differing definitions such as E-health, M-health, Tele-Play, and so on, into one term, Tele-mental health Play Therapy, stating that this would "reduce confusion and specifically convey the use of confidential, protected virtual platforms to provide psychological Play Therapy services from a distance". For those who identify as a play therapist and are registered, the more nuanced scaffolded definition provided in this chapter may prove useful (see Table 4.2). What is clear is that clinicians providing Tele-Play Therapy services must be a registered play therapist adhering to practice standards and ethical guidelines. Their professional practice should be informed by a model that is aligned with play therapy theory. Telecommunications practice includes clinical reasoning and therapeutic goals, both informed by the online mode of delivery. In some countries, maintaining registration as a play therapist requires a minimum number of clinical and supervision hours; the authors recommend clinical supervision for Tele-Play Therapy practice to ensure the scope of practice is maintained and clinical reasoning is exercised.

Tele-Filial Therapy

Filial Therapy includes a child's caregivers as the active therapeutic agents for change within a systemic family play therapy intervention (Cornett and Bratton, 2015). Filial Therapy has the strongest treatment effect size of all play therapy modalities (Bratton et al., 2005). A meta-analysis of play therapy research affirmed the increased benefits for the inclusion of caregivers in children's therapeutic processes (Bratton and Lin, 2015). Filial Therapy is easily adaptable for use with telecommunications due to the caregivers being involved throughout the intervention. With a strong treatment effect and systemic benefits, Filial Therapy should be prioritised if assessed as a viable option. Tele-Filial Therapy can be described as a virtual form of Filial Therapy or telecommunications for Filial Therapy. As Tele-Filial Therapy is an emerging intervention, efficacy and comparability to traditional Filial Therapy practice methods are, at this stage, only hypothesised. The authors have both practised and supervised practice in Tele-Filial Therapy. Informed from these experiences, five takeaway messages stand out: 1) conduct a thorough assessment phase; 2) collaboratively treatment plan within clinical supervision; 3) be ready to flexibly adapt throughout the intervention; 4) practice humility when virtually entering a family's home; and 5) harness the therapeutic power of positive emotions, congruently, through laughter and humour.

Scaffolded telecommunications for play therapy

Telecommunications for each scaffolded level of play therapy practice will now be compared in Table 4.2. The "Therapeutic scaffolding during an ongoing crisis" table has been adapted for the purpose of this chapter (VanFleet and Mochi, 2015; Renshaw and Parson, 2020: para. 5). Adherence to: 1) APPTA's

Table 4.2 Scaffolded telecommunications for play therapy.

Level of telecommunications for play therapy	Type of therapeutic activity or intervention	Focus of activity or intervention	Level of systemic support required
Tele-Play	Playful engagement through activities and games. Cultural consideration is required in choice of toys, resources, and games. As part of a remote intervention, activities are supported by the play therapist. Tele-Play sessions and recommendations should be recorded in clinical documentation.	Developmentally normative and engaging, playful and fun activities. These sessions may provide a platform for the practitioner to support familial relationships and identify needs. A safe and available environment is essential in the provision of normative play activities.	Tele-Play sessions are supported by the Play Therapist consulting with caregivers to facilitate the provision of normative playful activities for children. Consultation may also occur with service providers and community organisations within the child and family's system of support.
Tele-Health	Therapeutic alliance development and maintenance facilitated by regularly scheduled Tele-Health sessions between the play therapist and caregivers. As part of Tele-Health, parent support may be provided to prepare for parental facilitation of developmentally appropriate playful family activities and games. Cultural considerations essential. Tele-Health sessions and recommendations should be recorded using clinical documentation.	To alleviate parental stress, develop parenting skills and coping strategies, provide an opportunity for reflection and problem solving, build familial resilience, support the development of family relationships and opportunities for ongoing assessment of needs.	Tele-Health sessions between the play therapist and caregivers provide therapeutic consultation and support to the wider family system. The play therapist offers Tele-Health appointments to caregivers to support Tele-Play, Tele-Play Therapy, or Tele-Filial Therapy for children.

Tele-Play Therapy	The timing of remote interventions for individuals, families, or communities should be informed by best practice. The play therapist should only offer models of play therapy practice that are within their scope of practice. The Play Therapy Dimensions Model (PTDM) (Yasenik and Gardner, 2012) is a useful framework to inform an integrative humanistic stance to remote Play Therapy interventions. Models that inform an integrative approach could include: Humanistic Play Therapy (HPT), Child-Centred Play Therapy (CCPT), Prescriptive Play Therapy, directive approaches, Solution-Focused Play Therapy (SFPT), and Cognitive Behavioural Play Therapy (CBPT), and other models of Play Therapy practice.	Tele-Play Therapy interventions to child clients, families, and community organisations support psycho-social and emotional wellbeing. When needed, advocate for additional psychoeducational resources and activities for children that may be facilitated by the family. Link families and organisations with suitable resources that are complementary to the intervention.	Tele-Play Therapy sessions with children and adolescents are facilitated by the play therapist in consultation with caregivers. Consultation may also occur with other service providers and community organisations within the child and family's system of support.
Tele-Filial Therapy	Wherever appropriate and feasible select remote interventions with the strongest treatment effect. In play therapy, these interventions include the children and family, such as Filial Therapy (FT), Child–Parent Relationship Therapy (CPRT), and other systemic models of play therapy practice. The Play Therapist should only offer systemic models of practice that are within their scope of practice.	Tele-Filial Therapy interventions work within family systems to support children's psycho-social and emotional wellbeing through special play times with their own caregivers. Caregiver skills training and ongoing psychoeducation are embedded throughout the intervention. Ensure that families are well supported throughout a virtual intervention by friends, extended family, and other services such as schools, medical, or local community-based organisations.	Tele-Filial Therapy sessions with families are facilitated by the play therapist in consultation with caregivers. Consultation may also occur with other service providers and community organisations within the family's system of support.

Clinical Competencies and Practice Standards (APPTA, 2014b); 2) APPTA Guidelines for Ethical Play Therapy Practice (APPTA, 2020a); and 3) APPTA Personal Qualities (APPTA, 2020b) or other relevant play therapy industry guidance for the clinician's Country, State, Territory, or Region is advised across all levels of the table.

Guiding principles

In 2019, Parson, Renshaw, and Hurt proposed draft guidelines for therapeutic text messaging (RxTxT). These guidelines have been updated and extended for the purpose of this chapter (Parson et al., 2019: 76).

Guidelines for telecommunications in play therapy

1   Adhere to ethical principles when incorporating telecommunications into play therapy practice.
2   Assess the suitability of telecommunications with each client and family.
3   Obtain consent to incorporate telecommunications into the play therapy intervention from the caregiver and assent from the client.
4   Ensure confidentiality/digital security is carefully planned for each intervention.
5   Develop an emergency response protocol with the client and caregiver.
6   Establish boundaries for technology use within the therapeutic relationship.
7   Record use of technology in clinical notes, including interactions.
8   Store e-interactions securely.
9   Comply with data security laws in your country and state/authority.
10 Sit with any drafted e-messages and hold them before sending.

Contraindications for telecommunications in play therapy

Potential contraindications for the use of telecommunications in play therapy are a vital consideration for all persons involved in the intervention, i.e. the play therapist, the clinical supervisor/s, the child, and their family.

1   Not all persons involved in the intervention wish to participate.
2   Not all persons involved in the intervention feel they have the capacity for the inclusion of telecommunications at this time.
3   The caregivers do not currently have enough support in the context of the family constellation.
4   The environment is not physiologically, psychologically, or technologically safe.
5   Not all persons involved in the intervention have sufficient resources to utilise telecommunications – i.e. internet connectivity and competing demands on technology resources.

6   There is not a contained and private space in the home, and/or there is not sufficient access to toys and play resources.
7   The play therapist does not have emergency contact details for the family or emergency contact numbers do not work whilst engaged in therapy sessions, or an alternate method of communication between the caregivers and the therapist has not been established.

Preparation of the three environments

For Tele-Play Therapy practice to occur, the three environments must be prepared. The therapist will consider the circumstances and context for themselves, the client, and their connectivity within the virtual world.

Practitioner

The play therapy clinician will review their surroundings and set up the therapeutic space to engage the client. Two important aspects are the field of vision and audibility. Consideration of a virtual background has benefits and limitations. If you choose a virtual background, it could be a blurred background, or an alternative image or photograph may be used. Some clinicians have taken photographs of their Play Therapy room shelves displaying familiar toys (L. Yasenik, "Personal Communication", 7 May 2020). Whilst the virtual background may provide privacy and a consistent staging for play therapy sessions, it may inhibit a clear view if you want to show a client a toy or artefact through the camera.

Have the space to move from a seated position with the clients having only your head and shoulder view, to a standing position where the client can see whole-body movements for dance and role-play activities. Consideration is given to art and craft materials, puppets, and some of the usual toys found in the playroom. Miniatures and other artefacts should be readily available within the room and within easy reach so that you maintain an on-camera presence. Consideration for movement could also include a second camera to pan out the field of vision for the whole room or floor activities.

The Tele-Play Therapy space should have sounds that are only meant for the client's ears, removing any extraneous noises, e.g. family members talking, background TV or radio, pets, music, or other household noises. Therefore, setting up the practitioner's therapeutic space in a home office requires consideration of all family members to ensure a confidential, safe, and quiet space.

Client

Attention to the client's environment is just as important as the practitioner's surroundings. Converse with the parent to set the scene in readiness for the client with toys, art and craft materials, or specific online games or apps.

Instructing the parent to guide their child in setting up the space appropriately, in the use of the meeting technology or any other games or apps, may require a practise session initially with the parent and then with the child and parent before engaging in individual Tele-Play Therapy. Having an alternative means of communication with the parent for technological issues is important in reducing disconnection from the session.

Interconnected virtual settings

There may be additional costs in setting up an efficient and streamlined Tele-Play Therapy service. Having a quality computer with an integrated camera or second webcam source and a high-quality microphone or headset is important because the visual and sound quality will help facilitate the therapeutic relationship. Consideration of the internet service, connected to Wi-Fi or wired directly to the router, may impact internet stability and speed. It is also important to understand the viability of the client's internet service and if they can or cannot maintain live-video streaming. It may be worthwhile consulting an expert in telecommunications to assess specific needs.

Common digital acronyms used by children and adolescents:

- AFK – Away from keyboard
- BAK – Back at keyboard
- BRB – Be right back
- BTW – By the way
- CU – See you
- HTH – Hope this helps
- IDK – I don't know
- JK – Just kidding
- LOL – Laughing out loud
- ROFL – Rolling on floor laughing
- SUS – Suspicious
- TQ/THX – Thank you
- TYT – Take your time
- WTH – What the heck

See also www.smart-words.org/abbreviations.

Telecommunication practice considerations

When preparing to incorporate telecommunications into play therapy practice, there are logistical considerations prior to commencing practice. Five practice considerations have been identified and will be detailed in the scaffolded order: 1) scope of professional practice; 2) ethico-legal considerations; 3) technological equity; 4) software; and 5) financial transactions.

Scope of professional practice

Scope of professional practice is the foundational telecommunications consideration. The Play Therapy Hourglass (Figure 4.2) can assist clinicians to reflect on their telecommunications scope of practice. Scope of professional practice must be considered within one's primary discipline, play therapy practice, as well as the safe and effective use of digital technologies. Play therapists consider online training opportunities and additional supervision with more experienced Tele-Play Therapy practitioners.

Ethico-legal considerations

Next, there are several ethico-legal considerations to work through to prepare for commencing telecommunications work in play therapy. Four factors that are key to ensuring adherence to ethico-legal considerations are outlined, namely, license and/or registration, insurance, data protection compliance, and consent and privacy.

License and/or registration

First, ensure the currency of your license and/or registration to practice play therapy is maintained and allows for telecommunications practice. Licensing and registration bodies provide information on practice activities covered under their scope of practice. They may advise you on the legal requirements pertaining to remote Tele-Health service provision (Gilbertson, 2020).

Insurance

Next, verify with your insurance company that telecommunications practice is covered under your Professional Indemnity Insurance policy. Policies typically cover the specified geographical area for all activities listed on the schedule. This means that play therapists who work in a clinical setting (i.e. the physical playroom) are covered in the same way when working in an alternate location (i.e. virtually). A key factor is that clinical practice is covered when a clinician works within the scope of their registration. Some policies provide worldwide coverage but may exclude some countries (i.e. USA and Canada) which may require additional premiums.

Data protection compliance

Patient data protection is set by individual countries and healthcare practitioners adhere to the relevant legislation. To provide a few examples, in the USA, this is the Health Insurance Portability and Accountability Act (HIPAA), in the United Kingdom (UK) the General Data Protection Regulation, and in Australia the Privacy Act 1988 (Privacy Act) (Gilbertson, 2020). It is recommended that play therapists know and adhere to their country of practice data protection protocols. Adherence to best practice standards when internationally using telecommunications should include the country of practice and extend to the country of the client.

Consent and privacy

Adaptation of consent forms needs to be considered in relation to the virtual world and if all or part of the session is recorded in any way, including screenshots of artefacts (Gilbertson, 2020). It is sound practice to obtain consent and assent from both the parent and the child within sessions. As mentioned earlier, there is a need to consider the Tele-Play Therapy space including consideration of privacy for all parties.

Technological equity

Third, technological accessibility is a decisive factor when considering incorporating telecommunications into play therapy practice. Technological equity refers to inequalities in access to or functional use of telecommunication resources. Technological equity should be considered for all Tele-Play Therapy referrals. Tele-Play Therapy may not be suitable or accessible to all children and families. Careful discussion and assessment will aid in clinical reasoning for case planning. Three factors that are crucial for technological equity include geographical location, socioeconomic factors, and disability or health conditions.

Geographical location

Geographical location can limit internet connectivity, which may mean that HIPAA-compliant video-conferencing software platforms cannot be consistently used. When practising in geographically remote locations or in areas with poor connectivity, telephone communication may be another telecommunications option that is HIPAA compliant. However, Tele-Play Therapy can be limited if exclusively using a telephone as only verbal communication is possible. For this reason, clinicians may need to consider other telecommunication methods that allow for both verbal and non-verbal communication exchanges. During the Covid-19 pandemic, the HIPAA waiver allowed Tele-Health providers, including mental health clinicians to use more readily available video and chat apps, i.e. FaceTime or Facebook Messenger. This waiver did not extend to public-facing communication applications, i.e. Facebook or TikTok. Easily accessible telecommunication methods should be factored into interventions to pre-emptively plan for interruptions in connectivity.

Socioeconomic factors

Socioeconomic factors can limit telecommunications in two ways: 1) access to suitable hardware such as devices and software and 2) internet accessibility and stability of the connection. A 2017 study examining the socioeconomic *digital divide* found that technology was accessed by young people in both higher and lower socioeconomic neighbourhoods; however, differences appeared in how technology was accessed and engaged with (Harris et al., 2017). Higher socioeconomic factors indicated that technology was accessed via computers, whereas lower socioeconomic factors showed the technology was used via mobile phones, gaming consoles, and the television (Harris et al., 2017). These findings are useful when planning Tele-Play Therapy interventions. Explorative conversations about what telecommunications devices the family has access to (i.e. desktop computer, laptop, tablets, mobile phones) and how they access the internet (i.e. mobile phone data [3G, 4G, or 5G], Wi-Fi, broadband, cable) and the stability and reliability of their internet connectivity underpin the successful use of telecommunications for play therapy.

Disability or health conditions

Disability or health conditions should be carefully considered when planning the use of telecommunications in play therapy. Collaborative assessment with the caregivers of the current physical, sensory, and cognitive abilities of the child contributes to the process of ensuring optimal intervention accessibility. Bunyi et al. (2021: para. 6) acknowledged the need for accessibility and digital accessibility to be defined with adequate nuance, especially regarding digital mental health interventions, they stated that:

> For a resource to be most accessible, it must be able to be used by a person with a disability for the same purpose, the same effectiveness, and with a similar amount of time and effort as someone who is non-disabled. . . . In the context of the digital world, accessibility means that a website or tool is built with content and design that is understandable and navigable with or without assistive technologies.

Caregivers and sometimes even the child clients themselves (depending on age and abilities) can advise on individualised digital accessibility for suitable telecommunications in play therapy interventions. Play therapists are well positioned to recognise and acknowledge the family's expertise, learning from the family in a congruent manner.

Software

Software considerations are crucial in preparation for commencing telecommunication work in play therapy. Three factors to consider include choosing an online software platform, suitable applications (Apps) that may be free or require an investment purchase, and emerging software options such as Virtual Reality (VR).

Online platforms

Currently, there is a choice of suitable online software platforms. Considering the different teleconferencing software platforms and choosing the one that is most suitable for the therapeutic interventions you offer are paramount. Of the more frequently used and well-known teleconferencing software platforms, only three currently meet HIPAA regulations: 1) Zoom for Healthcare; 2) Microsoft Teams can be used stand alone or as part of the Microsoft Cloud healthcare for documentation; and 3) GoTo For Healthcare which includes GoToMeeting and GoToConnect. There is also a wide range of HIPAA-compliant video-conferencing software platforms designed especially for healthcare practice such as Doxy.me, VSee, SimplePractice Telehealth, and RingCentral for HealthCare, and some designed especially for mental health such as Thera-LINK. Of note, Doxy.me is currently the only free HIPAA-compliant teleconferencing software platform. This information will of course be subject to change over time, so regularly check to ensure your chosen teleconferencing software platform meets the data protection regulations that apply to your practice.

Applications (Apps)

Applications are often abbreviated to *Apps* and have mostly replaced the term *programs*. Apps refer to software that is installed on a device or accessed on a website. Suitable Apps for telecommunications play therapy interventions facilitate interactions between the therapist and the client, including the use of the whiteboard to draw and playing simple games such as tic tac toe, scribble, and copy what I draw or as directed by the child.

A range of freely available apps are available via the Oaklander Training website on the following links:

- Sandtray App
- Dollhouse App
- Puppet App
- Projective cards App

A paid version of a more sophisticated app is the *Virtual Sandtray App* (VSA). The authors have used this with clients and found that children and adolescents enjoy the functions that create movement in some of the characters, such as the dragon, and objects such as magic or fire. Additionally, the environmental options help to set a background scene to create a more expansive tone and may provide information regarding the clients' affect.

Virtual reality (VR)

The rapidly changing environment in the digital world is the emerging and immersive experiences that VR can offer. The field of paediatric mental health is starting to explore and research the inclusion of VR into interventions in both the physical clinical space and the virtual environment. VR can provide children with simulated experiences that may be like or unlike the real world. VR can be a virtual space to meet and chat using VR Chat. VR is currently an expensive inclusion into telecommunications for play therapy, so technological equity should be considered. However, for families that have access to VR headsets, several software apps may be used for therapeutic purposes. For specific training and supervision in immersive VR and play therapy, it may be wise to undertake training to become proficient in the use of VR in the first instance (for example, see *Dr Jessica Stone's* website www.jessicastonephd.com). Further studies are being undertaken in the field of VR and play therapy (see researchers Jingyuan (Jeffrey) Li and Jonathan Aitken www.jli.design/thesis2022).

Financial transactions

It is important to secure financial consent for Tele-Play Therapy interventions prior to the commencement of the service. Informed financial consent includes an agreement on the frequency of payments (i.e. after each session, fortnightly, monthly), the method of invoicing (i.e. postal, email, or business software), and the method of payment (i.e. cheque, bank transfer, accounting software online payment). Clinicians should also include a clause in their financial consent documentation on non-attendance and non-payment protocol.

Summary

In Section 1, the principles of Tele-Play Therapy were comprehensively summarised using four main categories, namely: telecommunications for play therapy, guiding principles, the three environments, and practice considerations. Figure 4.3 provides a visual summation of Section 1. In Section 2, a composite case example illustrates a Tele-Play Therapy intervention.

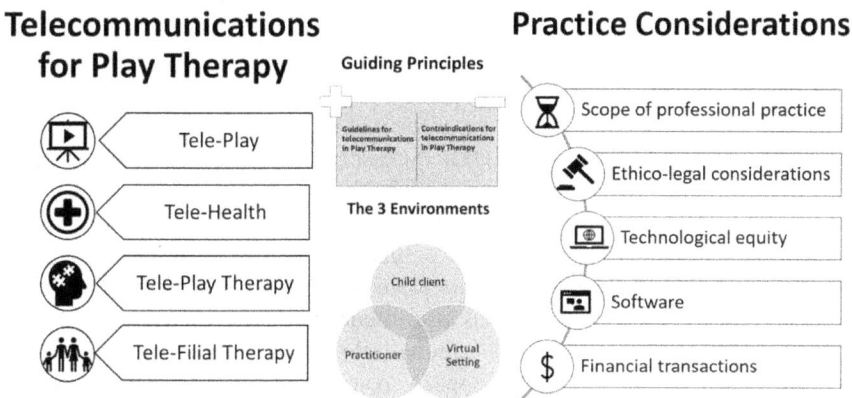

Figure 4.3 Principles of Tele-Play Therapy.

Section 2: a case study

Introducing Henry

Henry, an 8-year-old boy, was referred to play therapy just when the world was hearing about the Covid-19 pandemic. Henry's psychologist recommended play therapy as his social skills and play abilities were less mature compared to his chronological peers. He had low self-esteem and low affect. An initial intake, assessment, and two sessions were undertaken in person prior to a declared public health order in the Australian state of Victoria, limiting face-to-face contact and encouraging online interventions wherever possible. Social restrictions meant that play therapy in the traditional playroom swiftly moved into an online platform.

Family constellation

Henry comes from a culturally diverse family with his mother originally from Albania and his father describing himself as European Australian. Henry's parents separated two and a half years prior, and he resides with his mother and his 11-year-old brother, Simon. Henry had alternate weekends with his father, whereas Simon has no contact with his biological father. Henry's father and current partner have a 2-year-old daughter and another baby on the way. Henry and Simon have frequent Skype calls to their maternal grandparents in Albania. Henry also had a feline friend called Kenny the Kat, and he often expresses how much he loves Kenny and how much he hated school.

Description of child

Henry was above average in his height and weight, compared with his peers. His speech was at times difficult to understand. He was also seeing a speech pathologist. He came into the playroom a little nervous at first, but this was soon replaced with a smile and an eagerness to return to play therapy.

Assessments

The first assessment undertaken was informed by the Pretend Play Enjoyment Developmental Checklist (PPE-DC) (Stagnitti, 2017), which is an observational assessment used to understand Henry's play ability. I was interested in understanding how long Henry could enjoy and sustain play and focus his attention, how far he could extend or elaborate on his play sequences and actions, and how he could problem solve within play and engage in social interactions. I understood from this assessment that Henry struggled to sustain play and elaborate on storylines; he spoke little, but he did seem to enjoy playing with the toys and exploring the space created. This assessment also provided me with insights to plan and consider play interventions (Parson et al., 2020b).

The next projective assessment was the House-Tree-Person (Buck, 1948; Malchiodi, 1998). The therapist asks the client to draw a picture of a house, a tree, and a person, and Henry could choose to use one large piece of paper or three pieces. He chose one large piece, and after he completed the drawing, some questions were asked to describe the images. This type of projective assessment was used within a humanistic play therapy stance to gain insights into how Henry thought and felt about himself and his home. His simple drawing provided information about how he felt about his ability to draw, which was limited. He scribbled over the drawing of the person's face and said, "it's not very good" and "I can't draw". I noted how he approached the drawing activity and that it was quite haphazard, jumping from one area of the paper to another and then back again.

Clinical setting

To commence, the traditional playroom was used for the intake and assessment phase, which showed a full range of toys and expressive play materials. I suspected that this face-to-face contact made the transition to the Tele-Play and subsequent Tele-Play Therapy environment a little easier. However, I had not undertaken individual child play therapy online before, only Tele-Filial Therapy. I needed to upskill rapidly and sought additional supervision. I was ready to commence online Tele-Play, and once I had the opportunity to gauge the therapeutic interactions, in the context of the global pandemic crisis, I then transitioned to Tele-Play Therapy in alignment with Henry's readiness.

Transitioning from face-to-face to the virtual world

Setting up for the online Tele-Play session, I consulted with my supervisor and devised a clinical plan to have a range of more directive activities available. My home office became a resource with thoughtfully positioned play materials and easy-to-access pens, pencils, paper, cards, other stationery products, scissors, puppets, miniatures, and electronic resources such as my smartphone and iPad. My computer desk was positioned with two separate cameras and a Bluetooth headset – so I could move around the office. One of the cameras was framed for the sitting position, whereas the other camera was framed to view the mat on the floor. This enabled mirroring of my play area with the child's play space.

Like many play therapists at the time, I too was initially nervous about "doing" play therapy online. However, I reviewed my skills and knew that I was very capable of teaching online, so I prepared to start with Tele-Play to connect and build relational rapport with Henry in a playful way. But first I had to ensure that his home environment was supportive within the context of his family.

Parental support and phone contact

Initially, a planning session meeting was arranged with Henry's Mum to discuss the optimal space, resources, and guidelines to engage in home-based Tele-Play and ensure that Henry had a private space, free of interruptions from other members of the family or potential visitors. I wanted to ensure that Henry felt free to express himself in the way that he wanted to. I initially thought that Tele-Play would be holding the space and building the therapeutic relationship in the first instance.

Henry's Mum explained at intake that he was interested in Pokémon cards, Hot Wheels toy racing cars, soft plush toys, and Stikeez. Stikeez are small free give-away toys that were created to personify grocery items found at the store; examples include vegetables and fruits, cheese, fish, and yoghurt to name a few. They have a suction base to help them stand (or stick) to another surface. Henry collected and swapped his Stikeez with his friends at school. They were also perfect to use in Tele-Play because they could be tilted to show on camera. We devised a plan to ensure that some of these toys and others were available during our play sessions.

The consent form was revised, updated, and signed to engage in Tele-Play Therapy. We discussed the platform of Zoom and trialled it before the session. We confirmed mobile phone numbers for text messaging and phone calls, and I ensured that Mum was aware of the need for her to be available during Tele-Play Therapy sessions to support Henry as required.

Resources for Tele-Play Therapy

I sent a special play pack to Henry's mother with instructions that this was for exclusive use within the play sessions. This included a range of expressive arts resources such as coloured paper, pencils, felt-tip pens, crayons, paper scissors, sticky tape, eraser, sharpener, pipe cleaners, pom-poms, glue, and so on. I sent another container to collect junk that could be used for loose parts and creative play, buttons, small boxes, jars, stones, sticks, pinecones, and other natural objects. I also had similar resources in my home office to mirror activities. Another empty container was provided for Henry and his Mum to select a range of toys that may be suitable for playing within sessions – these items included his beloved cars and soft toys. In this situation, we decided that items in this container could be included in and outside of the Tele-Play sessions.

Let's play . . . online

For the first couple of sessions, Henry and I sat at the desk and went through the play kits and containers, and we checked out what we could see in each other's background. We played eye-spy looking at the limited space through the screen and noticing things in our fields of vision. We moved our cameras around so that we could show each other the rooms we were in and all the toys and play materials. This was when I decided to have a second camera, so I could toggle between the desk camera and the floor. Henry liked to play on the floor, and I wanted to mirror his positioning. Henry had a laptop that could be easily repositioned on or under his desk.

He showed me his Pokémon cards, and I made sure that I had researched some of the more common Pokémon characters, such as Evie, Squirtle, Bulbasaur, and Pikachu. I also had Rosie the puppet and a range of other puppets that would speak to Henry's cars and soft toy characters. On the fourth virtual session, Henry had already set up a scene ready to show me all his cars lined up along the wall and his soft toys ready for talking and tossing. We had moved into non-directive Tele-Play Therapy.

During these play sessions, he would also select a favourite song to play. He talked about Five Nights at Freddie's and Slenderman. I soon realised that Henry had access to a range of online content that seemed to be more appropriate for older-aged children and adolescents. Henry taught me how to draw Slenderman, Stikeez, Roblox, anime, and other characters. It was at these times that the therapeutic power of self-expression was evident and his self-esteem advanced.

Digital game play

One of Henry's most favourite pastimes was playing Roblox, which is an online multiplayer gaming app. He introduced me to many games including Adopt me, Brookhaven, Noob Train, and Freedraw 2. He also showed me how he had changed his avatars and he wanted to teach me how to create the same avatar. Within supervision, I discussed how to structure game playing. I decided that Roblox should only be played for 30 minutes of the 1-hour session, and Henry could not include others in our play sessions. We negotiated that we would create special avatars only for play therapy sessions!

I reflected on the various sessions using Roblox. I needed to become familiar with the functions and practice in between sessions, but it did provide me an entry point into Henry's world and use of these digital gaming apps. I noticed that in this world, he could truly lead the play and take me into uncharted play therapy territory, yet I was still able to maintain a humanistic stance.

Tele-Health – parent review meetings

Throughout the online Tele-Play Therapy, I organised meetings with Henry's Mum using telephone calls to check how Henry was going at home and school. She was often anxious about the pandemic and the ongoing periods of lockdown. She was home schooling two children as well as working and studying herself. Henry was "doing OK", and often these sessions were focused on Henry's mother's needs rather than Henry. However, it was important to support the family system at this time and check in with how the sessions were going and replenish any toys and resources as needed. Henry's Mum was also in personal therapy following the separation from her partner. Towards the end of six months, we decided that Tele-Filial Therapy would be ideal to enhance family relationships.

Tele-Filial Therapy

The Tele-Filial Therapy was contracted, and the first step was to undertake a Family Puppet Interview (FPI) (Irwin and Malloy, 1975). A box of puppets was sent as a kit to conduct the FPI, with a return paid postage. It was interesting to see the puppets come to life with the various family members projecting onto and through their puppets. Simon led the way and selected who should have which puppet. Henry was adamant that he should have the little blue monster puppet. Mum was given the shiny dragon puppet and she liked that it had sharp teeth. Simon had the spider and the crocodile puppet. Simon was the most talkative, and Mum withdrew a little to allow the children to play. The story line seemed chaotic and disjointed, yet they were constantly checking each other for the next moves. The selected animal puppets described a story of the spider who was wary of the crocodile and needed to get past the dragon and the blue monster to make a web on the other side of the pond. They discussed lots of ways for the spider to die, but the dragon was very protective of the spider and made sure that no harm would come to the spider.

This FPI provided insights to plan and prepare for Tele-Filial Therapy. In this case, the format was based on the Risë VanFleet (2005, 2012) Filial Therapy sequence.

Outcomes of Tele-Play Therapy

The case presentation of Henry has demonstrated a range of TPoPs through the virtual platform of Tele-Play, Tele-Health, Tele-Play Therapy, and Tele-Filial Therapy. Tele-Play provided the backdrop to continue to develop the therapeutic relationship, through self-expression, positive emotions, and empathy. Tele-Play Therapy offered opportunities for Henry to increase his personal strengths with a particular focus on building self-esteem, resiliency, creative problem solving, and promoting self-regulation. Throughout this stage, there were many moments of positive emotions with loud laughter echoing through my headset. Tele-Filial Therapy fostered emotional wellness by counterconditioning fears and enhancing the family's social relationships through catharsis, empathy, and attachment play. Like with traditional endings, virtual endings were considered and prepared for well in advance of the 'say goodbye' session as the final stage of the Tele-Filial Therapy sequence.

Conclusion

This chapter has contextualised the transcendence of traditional methods of play therapy service delivery into play therapy telecommunication inclusive practice. The principles of play therapy practice were detailed under the sub-categories of: 1) telecommunications for play therapy; 2) guiding principles; 3) preparation of the three environments; and 4) telecommunication practice considerations. Scaffolded telecommunications provide the potential for new models and methods of practising play therapy. Play therapists who undertake remote therapy using telecommunications will constantly acquire knowledge that will inform technological equity for all clinical cases. As the digital realm is continually updated, essential personal qualities include openness, a willingness to learn, and responsiveness. Fundamentally, remote interventions that can establish a therapeutic relationship and incorporate the therapeutic powers of play are an important option to consider when connecting with child clients and their families. Incorporating *digital technologies* into play therapy training programs is an important practice consideration for preparing the next generation of play therapists. As highlighted in the case of Henry and his family, the play therapist, as guided by the scaffolded approach to telecommunications practice in play therapy, enabled therapeutic work in a systemically collaboratively manner within the family system. Preparation and maintenance of the virtual therapeutic environment and adherence to both the guiding principles and practice considerations facilitated the activation of the therapeutic powers of play throughout the remote intervention.

References

APPTA (2014a) *Definition of play therapy*, available: https://appta.org.au/who-is-appta/.

APPTA (2014b) *Clinical competencies and practice standards*, available: https://appta.org.au/wp-content/uploads/2016/05/Clinical-competencies-and-Practice-Standards-ratified-at-AGM-Nov-2014.pdf.

APPTA (2020a) *APPTA Guidelines for ethical play therapy practice*, available: https://appta.org.au/wp-content/uploads/2021/02/Guidelines-for-Ethical-Practices.pdf.

APPTA (2020b) *Personal qualities*, available: https://appta.org.au/wp-content/uploads/2021/02/Personal-Qualities-.pdf.

Axline, V.M. (1964) *Dibs: In search of self*, New York, NY: Ballantine Books.

Axline, V.M. (1969) *Play therapy*, New York, NY: Ballantine Books.

Barak, A., Hen, L., Boniel-Nissim, M. and Shapira, N. (2008) 'A comprehensive review and a meta-analysis of the effectiveness of internet-based psychotherapeutic interventions', *Journal of Technology in Human Services*, 26(2/4), 109–160, Doi: 10.1080/15228830802094429.

Bratton, S.C. and Lin, Y. (2015) 'A meta-analytic review of child-centered play therapy approaches', *Journal of Counseling & Development*, 93, 45–58, Doi: 10.1002/j.1556-6676.2015.00180.x.

Bratton, S.C., Ray, D., Rhine, T. and Jones, L. (2005) 'The efficacy of play therapy with children: A meta-analytic review of treatment outcomes', *Professional Psychology, Research and Practice*, 4, 376, Doi: 10.1037/0735-7028.36.4.376.

Buck, J.N. (1948) 'The H-T-P test', *Journal of Clinical Psychology*, 4(2), 51–159, Doi: 10.1002/1097–4679(194804)4:2<151::AID-JCLP2270040203>3.0.CO;2-O.

Bunyi, J., Ringland, K.E. and Schueller, S.M. (2021) 'Accessibility and digital mental health: Considerations for more accessible and equitable mental health apps', *Frontiers in Digital Health*, 3, Doi: 10.3389/fdgth.2021.742196.

94 *Kate L. Renshaw and Judi A. Parson*

Cornett, N. and Bratton, S.C. (2015) 'A golden intervention: 50 years of research on filial therapy', *International Journal of Play Therapy*, 15(3), 119–133, Doi: 10.1037/a0039088.

Field, M.J. (1996) *Telemedicine: A guide to assessing telecommunications in health care*, Washington DC: National Academies Press.

Gilbertson, J. (2020) *Telemental health: The essential guide to providing successful online therapy*, Eau Claire, WI: PESI Publishing & Media.

Glazer, H. (2017) 'Play therapy in the digital age: Practice and training', in S.L., Brooke (ed.) *Combining the creative therapies with technology: Using social media and online counseling to treat clients*, Springfield: Charles C. Thomas, 25–33.

Harris, C., Straker, L. and Pollock, C. (2017) 'A socioeconomic related "digital divide" exists in how, not if, young people use computers', *PloS One*, 12(3), e0175011, Doi: 10.1371/journal.pone.0175011.

Hutton, D. (2004) 'Margaret lowenfeld's 'world technique', *Clinical Child Psychology and Psychiatry*, 9(4), 605–612, Doi: 10.1177/1359104504046164.

Irwin, E.C. and Malloy, E.S. (1975) 'Family puppet interview', *Family Process*, 14(2), 179.

Maeder, A. and Smith, A.C. (2010) '*Global telehealth*', selected papers from Global Tele-health 2010 (GT2010): 15th International Conference of the International Society for Telemedicine and eHealth and 1st National Conference of the Australasian Telehealth Society, Amsterdam: IOS Press.

Malchiodi, C.A. (1998) *Understanding children's drawings*, ProQuest Ebook Central, available: https://ebookcentral.proquest.com.

Mochi, C. and VanFleet, R. (2009) 'Roles play therapists play: Post-disaster engagement and empowerment of survivors', *Play Therapy*, 4(4), 16–18, available: www.play-therapy.com/images_prof/MochiVanFleetPTarticle.pdf.

Moustakas, C. (1959) *Psychotherapy with children*, New York, NY: Harper & Row.

Mullen, J.A. (2021) 'TelePlay therapy', in L., Fazio-Griffith and R., Marino (eds.) *Techniques and interventions for play therapy and clinical supervision*, Hershey, PA: IGI Global, 252–270. Information Science Reference (Advances in psychology, mental health, and behavioral studies (APMHBS) book series).

Parson, J. and Hickson, S. (2016) *Online interactive supervision for play therapy*, British Association of Play Therapists conference, Aston Centre. Birmingham, UK, 24 June 2016.

Parson, J., Renshaw, K., and Zimmer, T. (2018). *Play therapy hourglass*, Deakin University Short course, Foundational Concepts and skills for Child Play Therapy, Deakin University Waterfront Campus, Geelong, Australia, November, 26–27.

Parson, J., Renshaw, K. and Hurt, A. (2019) 'RxTxT: Therapeutic texting', in J., Stone (ed.) *Integrating technology into modern therapies: A clinician's guide to developments and interventions*, Oxon: Routledge.

Parson, J., Renshaw, K., and Zimmer, T. (2020a). 'The Therapeutic Powers of Play', info-graphic. An earlier version is Parson, J. (2017) 'Puppet play therapy: Integrating Theory, Evidence and Action (ITEA)', presented at the International Play Therapy Study Group, Champneys at Forest Mere, England. June 18, Adapted from Schaefer, C.E. and Drewes, A.A. (2014) *The therapeutic powers of play: 20 core agents of change*, 2nd edn., Hoboken, NJ: Wiley.

Parson, J., Stagnitti, K., Dooley, B. and Renshaw, K. (2020b) 'Play ability', in J.A., Courtney (ed.) *Infant play therapy: Foundations, models, programs and practice*, New York, NY: Routledge, 53–66.

Renshaw, K. and Parson, J. (2020) *APPTA response to COVID-19 (Coronavirus)*, APPTA, available: https://appta.org.au/wp-content/uploads/2020/03/APPTA-Reponses-to-COVID-19-March-2020.pdf.

Renshaw, L.K. and Parson, J.A. (2021) 'It's a small world: Projective play', in E., Prendiville and J., Parson (eds.) *Clinical applications of the therapeutic powers of play: Case studies in child and adolescent psychotherapy*, London: Routledge, 72–86.

Renshaw, K., Parson, J. and Hurt, A. (2015) 'RxTxT: Engaging adolescents with avoidant attachment behaviours by therapeutic texting', conference paper, *Australasia Pacific Play Therapy Association*, Towards the future, Melbourne, 10 August 2015.

Rogers, C.R. (1957) 'Necessary and sufficient conditions of therapeutic personality change', *Journal of Consulting Psychology*, 21, 95–103.

Schaefer, C.E. and Drewes, A.A. (2014) *The therapeutic powers of play: 20 core agents of change*, 2nd edn., Hoboken: John Wiley & Sons, Inc.

Stagnitti, K. (2017) *Pretend play enjoyment developmental checklist*, Melbourne: Learn to Play.

Stone, J. (2019) *Integrating technology into modern therapies: A clinician's guide to developments and interventions*, New York, NY: Routledge.

Stone, J. (2020) *Digital play therapy: A clinician's guide to comfort and competence*, New York, NY: Routledge.

Stone, J. (ed.) (2021) *Play therapy and telemental health: Foundations, populations, and interventions*, ProQuest Ebook Central, available: https://ebookcentral.proquest.com.

Turner, B.A. (2004) *H.G Wells' floor games. A father's account of play and its legacy of healing*, California: Temenos Press.

VanFleet, R. (2005) *Filial therapy: Strengthening parent-child relationships through play*, 2nd edn., Sarasota, Florida: Professional Resource Press.

VanFleet, R. (2012) *A parent's handbook of filial therapy. Building strong families with play*, 2nd edn., Boiling Springs: Play Therapy Press.

VanFleet, R. and Mochi, C. (2015) 'Enhancing resilience through play therapy with child and family survivors of mass trauma', in S., Goldstein, R.B., Brooks and D.A., Crenshaw (eds.) *Play therapy interventions to enhance resilience*, New York, NY: The Guilford Press, 168–193.

Wells, H.G. (1911) *Floor games*, London: Frank Palmer.

Winnicott, D.W. (1965) *The maturational processes and the facilitating environment: Studies in the theory of emotional development*, London: Hogarth.

Winnicott, D.W. (1971) *Playing and reality*, London: Tavistock Publications.

Yasenik, L. and Gardner, K. (2012) *Play therapy dimensions model: A decision-making guide for integrative play therapists*, 2nd edn., London: Jessica Kingsley Publishers.

5 Learn to Play Therapy in high-risk countries

The example of Nigeria

Claudio Mochi and Karen Stagnitti

The authors describe the key role of teachers and other local professionals in applying play and Play Therapy to: create an optimal learning environment; foster fundamental skills in children such as narrative language ability, self-regulation, and emotional-social competence; and support children in reaching their potential and overcoming psychosocial problems. The gradual progression from introductory activities to more specialised activities is also presented highlighting the importance of adapting daily practice to identified needs. Case studies are provided to bring the content "alive" and illustrate the concrete application of the Learn to Play approach.

The beauty of nature and the incredible playfulness of children remind us we are far from the ongoing conflict in the North of Nigeria and from the tough political clashes in the other Nigerian States. At first sight, the villages served by the project offered a rare picture of children playing in open spaces, enjoying nature, distant from the dangers and the chaos of the biggest cities.

The project "Developing Play Together" was created and implemented in the Regions of Ikeduru and Mbaise in the Southern State of Imo, Nigeria. In this area, the presence of foreigners is extremely rare as there are no international associations apart from the Italian SOSolidarietà ("SOS"). SOS in collaboration with the Nigerian local partner, the Sisters of the Most Precious Blood, targeted a restricted area and built a clinic providing medical support services. Through the years, they also developed programs to provide basic needs to vulnerable families and facilitated access to schools for many children whose families could not afford private schooling or even basic school supplies. SOS volunteers observed generations of children and, with deeper involvement, concluded that something more was needed, particularly for facilitating their development. They reported children appeared "well behaved", especially with adults, but they also observed children were somehow apathetic, rigid, easily distracted, at times fearful, and with a lot of academic difficulties.

Nigeria is the most populated African country. In 2019 on the Human Development Index (1), the country reached the position of 167 out of 189 recognised states and territories (UNDP, 2019: 2). According to the same report, the last 20 years have marked an improvement in many dimensions with an increase of 15.9% in the index (op. cit.). Many measures such as life

DOI: 10.4324/9781003252375-6

expectancy have grown, but the inequality across the country increased to 35.9%. The level of crisis in the country is considered "very high" according to the INFORM Index (IASC and EC, 2021). The Multidimensional Poverty Index that measures deprivation in health education and living conditions reports that a minority of the population is above the poverty line (0.5%) and one person in two (53.9%) suffers the highest level of deprivation (op. cit.: 5).

Even though Ikeduru and Mbaise are not involved in armed hostilities, the population has to deal with deprivation and difficulties on a daily basis. Shootings, kidnappings, and child abuse are not regular events, but they do occur. The political tension takes up considerable space in the worries of adults. The vast majority of children and youth live in very poor conditions, often malnourished and affected by malaria. Cases of HIV are present, access to health services is poor, and there is no social welfare (SOS and INA, 2012).

Apart from a few exceptions, families do not have immediate availability of water, generators for electricity, or any other appliances that can ease the daily workload. Most adults have long days of work in the fields and many children to manage. As Elkind (1987: xii) would say, at the end of the day, parents "have few resources left to cope with the unending needs of children". Most households have to rely on children to carry out different house chores and errands. Children at a very young age have to learn a variety of skills and have few other enriching opportunities apart from the school setting. In contrast with researchers (Garbarino, 1999; Dunst et al., 2000; Masten, 2009) who advocate for a wide variety of everyday learning experiences to foster children's wellbeing and development, the opportunities that families and society can offer are restricted to community and religious ceremonies and football.

Project background

> Childhood is a protected niche in the social environment, a special time and place in the human life cycle, having a special claim on the community.
>
> (Garbarino, 1999)

Even before arriving in the region and meeting the children, we knew the context was a high-risk environment for their development. The way our brain organises and matures in response to the environment can make us very adaptable or vulnerable according to our experiences and, for children in particular, chronic levels of stress and scarcity of learning opportunities can affect a child's development and lifetime possibilities (Perry et al., 1995; Shore, 1997).

Semeroff and colleagues underlined that "cumulative effects from multiple risk factors increase the probability that development will be compromised" (1987: 343). According to their studies, the risk for children to have intellectual and social-emotional disturbance could reach a probability of 50% when four or five factors were combined. Considering the elements included in Semeroff et al.'s research, such as low family income and education, lack of social support, the presence of stressful events, parents' rigid perspectives, and large family size, the majority of children in the region were at risk and "24 times as likely to have IQs below 85 than low-risk children" (op. cit.). Even though the research was based on data collected from a different and more industrial context, Ikeduru and Mbaise were regions where there were combinations of many difficult conditions with restricted learning opportunities and weakened social support. The potential negative impact on a child's development was real.

The UNDP report (2019) indicates how slow and fragile the process is to improve certain conditions. Children, as developing individuals, have limited capacity to mediate the pressure of their contexts, and we could not change the most severe aspects of their reality. What we could do, in a relatively short time, was to potentiate those factors that can reduce children's vulnerability and foster their wellbeing. Garbarino (1998), for instance, pointed out seven "ameliorating factors that lead to pro-social and healthy adaptability": 1) actively trying to cope with stress, 2) cognitive competence, 3) experiences of self-efficacy and a corresponding self-confidence and positive self-esteem, 4) temperamental characteristics that favour active coping and positive relationships with others, 5) a stable emotional relationship with at least one parent or other reference person, 6) an open, supportive educational climate that encourages constructive coping with problems, and 7) social support from persons outside the family.

The project "Developing Play Together" was created with the purpose of enhancing individual and relational protecting factors in conjunction with a sustainable local support system as defined in Chapter 1. The organisations in the local system that we selected, together with local partners (including the Ministry of Education), consisted initially of five schools and a couple of associations. We all believed that expanding knowledge and abilities of the staff would be reflected in increased possibilities for children to develop relevant abilities and experience a more enriched environment (see Vygotsky, 1978).

The school environment and the need for play

> Fostering play classrooms for children from lower socioeconomic and high-risk environments is particularly important in order to build the foundation skills for learning that are missing.
>
> (Stagnitti, 2010: 145)

Before going into the details of the project, it is important to provide an introduction to the school context and the reasons that motivated and guided us to choose Learn to Play Therapy (LtP) and why this approach represented a turning point in our intervention.

The playgrounds of the schools in our project were quite vast. In this outside space, we were warmed and welcomed by the children's smiling faces as they ran around. The classes, on the contrary, were not ideal locations to work and learn. They were quite small and crowded with an average of 30 students and sometimes even 40 or 50 children in a class. Some classrooms had no walls or other physical separation and, in some cases, a big noisy hall would contain an entire elementary school with no less than 150 students. From kindergarten, children were engaged in rote academic learning with didactic teaching. For example, the teaching method was based on presenting the content and requesting children either to collectively repeat it or to complete the sentences teachers pronounced. The didactic teaching approach had few variations and, considering that classes continued for 5–7 hours each day, the level of energy required by teachers was huge. The participation from students was restricted to conforming to teachers' requests under a "strict" discipline. Discipline was often metered out by loud shouting, the use of a stick and in some cases bamboo canes. A commonly observed punishment saw children kneeling on the ground for a long time in front of the entire school. From the teachers' point of view, this method worked, as children completely observed the regulations even in the absence of supervision.

After the first round of school visits, we realised that teachers and students were highly dedicated. We also concluded that the children's learning experience at school could be expanded by offering alternatives for new learning opportunities within a safer and more pleasant context. In our meetings and training sessions, we were pleased to find groups of teachers, who were open and motivated on expanding their repertoire of relational skills and educational strategies. They were also keen on learning how to use the power of play to create a positive atmosphere, manage difficult situations, and promote learning.

The core of the project focused on training teachers in the progressive integration of new relational abilities and different play-based activities. After several months, the first 30 teachers were including a free play time lasting 20–30 minutes in their daily program. Inspired by the Filial Therapy model (Guerney, 1964; VanFleet and Guerney, 2003), teachers were using child-centred techniques to follow the children's interests and play initiatives. Considering the number of children, the restricted space, and the fact that many children had never seen some of the toys before, several adaptations to the original model had to be made. The overall experience worked well: children were happy and the atmosphere in the classes was gradually changing. Over time teachers started to generalise the child-centred abilities to facilitate their interactions. Children became more emotionally engaged and confident and more self-regulated in their play. The project was going to plan, except that children's pretend play abilities did not improve and "when a child's pretend play skills are poor, they begin school at-risk for failure because poor pretend play also reflects a child's lack of ability to sequentially think through a logical sequence of thought" (Stagnitti, 2010: 149).

For the majority of children, their play remained at the sensory-motor level with manipulation and experimentation of the play materials, stacking blocks, moving cars back and forth, and fighting with dolls. The magic moment when children start to "impose their meaning on the toys" in "their play" (Stagnitti,

2021: 11) did not arrive. Children in the elementary classes (that is, children aged 6–11 years) showed early pretend play ability at the 24 months level. When their play was not sensory and movement, the play scripts were related to everyday events, such as carrying babies on their back and washing clothes or performing short sequences of traditional dance. They frequently exchanged toys and play material, but social complex pretend play interactions were not observed. Even for the more advanced players, play did not "transcend reality" and was never "unpredictable" (Stagnitti, 2021: 12). The reference to the *Pretend Play Enjoyment Developmental Checklist* (Stagnitti, 2017) indicated that all children were at the very early stages of their pretend play.

Maybe we should not be surprised by the level of the children's pretend play since their environment had not stimulated such play and all children had experienced rigid formal schooling very early and intensely. We also knew that "asking children to perform academic tasks at early ages was potentially damaging" (Hartigan cited in Brooks, 2009: 9). All children displayed relevant life skills that many adolescents in other contexts would barely possess. At a very young age, they had responsibilities in their households, and at school, they were in charge of cleaning, organising materials in the classes, getting the water, managing the gardens, and taking care of younger children. They were refined players in traditional games and football, able to walk for great distances, but at the same time, had little experience in playful, pretend play interactions. Vygotsky (cited in Stagnitti, 2021: 18) "saw children's development being spurred by symbolic play with a more competent other". Children without these kinds of experiences missed important sources of imitation and the practice of all the processes that are involved when pretend play is shared. If "learning is a representation of experience" (Dewey cited in Elkind, 1987: 23), the children we met needed support in expanding their experiences starting from *recovering their lost play time* (see Chapter 3) with a present and competent adult (Stagnitti, 2021). We knew that, in line with this emerging need, adaptations had to be made, and we thought about introducing the LtP approach that "aims to develop the enjoyment and the ability in pretend play" and offers the possibility of "a continuum from groups in schools to one-to-one therapy" (op. cit.: 11).

I (Claudio) remember the first day we experimented with this approach in one class. Isabella Cassina and I were in a kindergarten class and, following the LtP process, we started at children's play level and applied the child-centred abilities in order to promote an atmosphere of safety. After a while, when we noticed that the children's play remained at the sensory-motor level, we decided to start engaging them in early pretend play by feeding our puppets with a spoon. We did not need to work hard to get the children's attention because they looked at us right away with stupor and curiosity and, after a moment of total enjoyment, they all wanted our puppets! Most of these young children probably believed that our puppets were special and could perform different actions from theirs. There was enthusiasm all around us. We kept feeding the characters and, in a short time, something happened: some children wanted to be included in the play and receive food themselves and, after some time, some others took over the role of the food provider.

Following the LtP approach, we introduced some variations in our sequence using other characters and having them drink from a glass instead of eating. Not all children joined this new form of play and many continued in manipulation and sensory-motor play. Nevertheless, the beauty of working with groups of children is that, very often, when one child understands a new possibility and starts his own pretend play, others will imitate him/her. We could see this approach working, and it was just a matter of time to reach all children in this new adventure.

In those early experiences, we realised how powerful it was to apply the "Learn to Play approach in schools" (Stagnitti, 2021). The children's exposure to alternative possibilities (that is, our modelling of pretend play actions using the play materials) opened up different positive scenarios, which changed the kind of play and the level of enjoyment in the interactions between children and the teachers. Pretend play has a fundamental importance for the development of future abilities and from that moment we confirmed the LtP approach as part of our project, with the intention for children and teachers to engage in "developing play together".

Pretend play across cultures

The play of children has been observed across cultures from around the world. These observations have been reported in books and journal articles by those with an interest in other cultures (for example, developmental psychologists, sociologists, anthropologists, and researchers). In this chapter, pretend play is the focus as it is core to the LtP approach. Pretend play is also known by other names such as imaginative play, make-believe play, representational play, or fantasy play. Pretend play is a unique form of play because it involves the imposition of meaning beyond the literal play space or play materials (Stagnitti, 2021). For example, the child may use objects in substitution for other objects (e.g. the box is a car), attribute properties to toys and play materials (e.g. the puppet is hungry), and reference absent objects (e.g. it's raining when there is no rain). Pretend play involves sustained symbolic thinking, the creation of a story in play, the involvement of a child in a role, and the decentring from self to impose emotions and feelings on toys such as dolls or puppets (Stagnitti, 2010). Pretend play can also be imposed on other types of play, for example, an obstacle course that is set up for gross motor (large muscle) play can become an adventure in a jungle (with balance beams being bridges over rivers and tunnels being caves).

So why is this type of play relevant to a project in schools in Nigeria? Pretend play has been linked to the abilities that a child needs to function within a school environment, such as narrative language ability (Nicolopoulou et al., 2010; Stagnitti and Lewis, 2015), metacognition, metacommunication, self-regulation, and emotional-social competence (Whitebread and O'Sullivan,

2012; Bodrova et al., 2013; de Haan et al., 2021; Richard et al., 2021). Optimal learning environments for children are context-driven rather than task-specific (Zosh et al., 2018). Playful contexts for learning provide environments where children learn best because learning is active (minds-on), engaged (not distracting), meaningful (transferred to outside of school), and occurs in socially interactive environments where there is joy (positive affect) and iteration (Zosh et al., 2018: 3). Positive affect or joy is an element of play (Eberle, 2014) and has been linked to increased executive functions, academic success, and brain flexibility (Zosh et al., 2018: 3). Iteration is a hallmark of play as children construct new knowledge based on hypothesis testing and revision of knowledge over time (Zosh et al., 2018). In a classroom, guided play (where the adult arranges a context for learning but the child directs the play within that context) has been found to be more effective for a child's learning than didactic teaching methods (op. cit.).

Pretend play ability has been observed in children in cross-cultural contexts (Haight et al., 1999). From 2 years of age, children understand the intentionality of pretend play (Rakoczy, 2008a), i.e. they understand the meaning in the play, share and create shared meaning with others (Creaghe et al., 2021). Rakoczy argued that this ability to collectively negotiate, the "we-intentionality" of the play, between the child and others "lays the foundation for the development of culture" (Rakoczy, 2008b: 506). A child's pretend play reflects their culture through the objects used in play (toys, objects, and absent objects), their play partners, their interactions with caregivers, and the stories in their play (Haight et al., 1999). In Haight et al.'s study, children from Irish American and Taiwanese families were observed and videoed in their home, twice for 2 hours, over the ages of 30, 36, and 48 months. Cross-culturally, the children's pretend play increased in complexity as they grew, with caregivers capitalising on a child's increased fluency in pretend play to show their child culturally appropriate social interactions. For example, some of the Taiwanese caregivers, in their play interactions with their child, were observed to demonstrate showing respect to a teacher by bowing (Haight et al., 1999). In essence, Haight et al. (1999) argued universal dimensions of pretend play to be: the use of objects and the social activity of the play; developmental dimensions were a child's increasing initiation and elaborateness of their play; and variable dimensions were culture-specific. In another study, the pretend play of Brazilian children across five different cultural groups showed that children in all groups engaged in pretend play with cultural variations in the content of their observed pretend play (Gosso et al., 2007). For example, object substitution (e.g. a lemon for soap) was more frequently observed among Indian girls, whereas role-play (e.g. being a mother or child) was more frequently observed in the Seashore and Mixed SES urban children groups (op. cit.).

In support of the literature on cross-cultural observations of children's development of pretend play, typically developing children were found to have increasingly elaborate spontaneous pretend play in Brazil (Lucisano et al., 2020), Taiwan (Lee et al., 2016), Iran (Dabiri Golchin et al., 2017), and Finland

(Tigerstied and Stagnitti, 2014). To be culturally responsive, changes to play materials and administration of the Child-Initiated Pretend Play Assessment were made for Australian Aboriginal children (Dender and Stagnitti, 2011, 2017). There is little reported research on African children and pretend play. This chapter adds to the literature.

Learn to play – what and how

Not all children develop the ability to pretend in play. This realisation led to Learn to Play Therapy (Stagnitti, 2021) which is the therapeutic use of play.

First, we shall explain this approach. Learn to Play Therapy aims to increase a child's ability to spontaneously initiate their own pretend play and understand the intentionality of the play. It was developed for children who struggle to engage in pretend play or social pretend play with peers. The theoretical underpinnings of this therapeutic approach are the child-centred approach as explained by Axline (1974), Vygotsky's view of mental development and play within the zone of proximal development (Vygotsky, 2016), and the neurobiological research on play. Several skills are the focus of Learn to Play Therapy which are: the ability to sequence pretend play actions; object substitution (using an object to represent something else in play, such as a block for a phone); play scripts (the stories in the play), doll/teddy/figurine play; role-play; and social pretend play (Stagnitti, 2021). Within each of these skills is layered a child's ability to understand the intentionality of the play with the ability to go beyond the literal by attributing properties to objects (e.g. the teddy is naughty), referring to absent objects (e.g. a child announced "it is raining"), sustaining symbolic thinking, and understanding the context of the play. In preparing developmentally appropriate play activities for children, one is always reminded to consider the child's culture by the thoughtful choice of toys and materials, colours, and understanding the social context of a child's everyday life (op. cit.).

For over 25 years, techniques that have proven to be effective within LtP are: repetition with variation, gaining the child's focused attention, challenging the child to higher levels of play, talking about the play as the child plays, choosing developmentally and culturally responsive play activities, and emotionally engaging the child in the joy and pleasure of play (Davidson and Stagnitti, 2021; Stagnitti, 2021).

Learn to play in classrooms

Children and adults are social beings, and the brain is socially gated (Hirsh-Pasek and Golinkoff, 2020). Pretend play is linked to a child's learning through research exploring narrative, literacy, and a child's socio-emotional wellbeing. Children who began formal schooling with low levels of pretend play ability were not ready to learn and were socially disconnected (Reynolds et al., 2011). When pretend play was embedded in classrooms and children were exposed to teachers guiding children in appropriate play activities throughout the week, the child's ability to pretend play grew and this was associated with an increase in narrative language, social competence, and grammar ability (Reynolds et al., 2011; Stagnitti et al., 2016). For children with IQs below 70, LtP was adapted for special school classrooms and after 22 weeks children were found to be more socially connected (O'Connor and Stagnitti, 2011). In another study, teachers reported a deeper engagement of children in learning and transfer of social skills into the home after seven months of implementing the LtP approach in their schools (Wadley and Stagnitti, 2020).

Project guidelines

The project lasted five years and over this time, progressively developed according to our field observations, feedback, and reflections from all partners. This project started because of the remarks of the SOS volunteers, the ability of partners to involve the first five schools, and the MAP (see Chapter 1) we "carried" with us. The project was based on the following three guidelines.

1   *Support schools in their primary role* of "providing enriched social and play experiences that children might not receive at home" (Elkind, 1987: 4). Schools are one of the most powerful supportive and adaptive systems created to "foster and protect human development" (Masten, 2009). Even in disadvantaged and high-risk contexts, school interventions have several advantages including "promoting and protective factors" in the "ordinary magic" of the class interactions (op. cit.). Schools are in a unique position to provide children with resources such as a safe context, structure, and guidance, co-regulation, learning material, and the stimulation of a child's emerging abilities. Schools represent a natural environment (Dunst et al., 2000) for children where, more than in any other context, it is possible to reach a large number of them (Drewes, 2001) and offer different levels of interventions including preventing problems, promoting abilities, and general development (Drewes, 2001; Peabody et al., 2010).

2   *Enhance teachers' and educators' capacities.* Professionals of the school environment are important community figures, who have a large impact directly and indirectly, in the lives of children. "Teachers can influence students' learning through actions, thought processes, and beliefs" (Stagnitti, 2010: 154). The "simple" improvement of the teacher–child relationship has a profound positive effect on children. Teachers trained in relational-building skills have the possibility to "impact students' social/emotional development, academic achievement, and classroom functioning" (Morrison and Pretz Helker, 2010: 182–183). As Andronico and Guerney (1967) suggest, teachers can be important agents of change in children; they can build an "open and supportive educational climate" (Garbarino, 1998) and create multiple occasions to help children develop abilities such as

self-confidence, self-efficacy, self-control, and social skills (Drewes, 2001; Post, 2001; Reddy, 2010).

In addition, teachers who have relational-building competence can better manage emotional or behavioural difficulties of children and feel less stressed (Morrison and Pretz Helker, 2010: 182). Compared with other interventions that involve external resources, building teachers' internal competence has the extra value of sustainability, especially when they teach several generations of children.

3 *Apply the powers of play* to enrich the quality of school interactions in order to provide a regular and more diverse context for growth and wellbeing. "Optimal brain development depends on healthy play experiences in early life" (Panksepp, 2010: 245) and, as Ginsburg (2007: 182) points out, "it contributes to the cognitive, physical, social, and emotional wellbeing of children and youth". In this project, play and play therapy skills and activities "serve as adjunct to the learning environment" offering "experiences that assist children in maximising the opportunities for learning" (Landreth cited in Drewes, 2001: 48), by providing multiple ways to improve relationships and foster wellbeing.

Project structure overview

When we realised the huge need to invest in pretend play, the project was strongly redefined and accordingly renamed "Developing Play Together". Initially, the project included five private schools and one centre for extra-curricular activities called "Happy Home" (HH). After the Secretary of Education of the Ikeduru Region agreed to the project, 60 teachers enrolled in the 120-hour training program. In the first 5 years, 1,600 children were reached.

School intervention

The entire project was developed and refined in different stages. Powers of play and relational abilities were used to offer children the following experiences:

a) *Safe and pleasant environment.* Teachers learnt how to structure a conducive learning environment using toys to teach and play rituals at different times of the day. They also generalised child-centred abilities, such as empathic listening and limit setting, to attend to children's behavioural and emotional needs without recurring to physical punishment. This facilitated more positive interactions between children and themselves.

b) *Pretend play practice.* On a daily basis, teachers using the "Learn to Play approach in schools" provided children with opportunities for pretend play experiences. Children could interact with each other using developmentally appropriate toys and play materials. Meanwhile, teachers and the project team assisted children to consolidate and extend pretend play skills.

c)   *Self-regulation experiences.* Together with free play, teachers introduced specific traditional and non-traditional structured activities to support children in practising self-regulation. Teachers were trained to co-regulate
children's level of activity, using calming activities to modulate the class's
enthusiasm, to stimulate attention and participation, and to reengage children when they were inattentive or bored. At the same time, teachers benefited from having more capacity to manage difficult situations and feeling
less stressed with a more engaged class.

d)   *Active participation in learning.* Another important component was using the
method we called "Play, Learn and Grow" (PLeG) to teach. Teachers were
supported to implement in their classes what they had experienced in our
training. PLeG aimed to create fun and more active participation in the
classes (Bodrova and Leong, 2006; Stagnitti, 2021). The main goal was to
engage students by using play and other expressive and creative modalities while introducing different topics. Then, children's active participation in learning was stimulated using a variety of interaction opportunities
where children worked and elaborated on the topic in smaller groups. This
modality offered children opportunities to learn through different creative
and expressive channels and allowed teachers to express and enhance their
own creativity in teaching.

Happy Home intervention

The second element of the project included HH, the after-school centre where
children from nearby villages could access activities free of charge. Before starting the project, the centre was a place for children to receive support with their
homework and enjoy recreational activities and medical interventions. HH
afforded the possibility to extend the school "play" time with the advantage of
bigger spaces, non-academic pressure, and smaller groups.

Four educators were in charge of a 3-hour program from Monday to Friday
for children aged 3–17 years. One of the educators was responsible for kindergarten and junior school and one other for junior high school. These two
educators have been the pillar of the project. They were responsible for at least
150 children in the afternoon and 60 teachers during the whole school year.
We worked together in every phase of the project; we shared a lot of thinking
and learnt from each other. These educators experienced more training with
shared activities. They received extra individual supervision consolidating their
skills. Over time, they became a valuable resource who supported and supervised all other teachers.

The HH program was an afternoon program that offered extra opportunities
for fun and learning with two additional components: provide more specific
support and consolidate the support system. There were minor variations, but
the general structure consisted of three parts, adjusted for different age groups.
There was a time for recreation and free play in the courtyard. As in the school,
this was child-centred oriented and then shifted to LtP. The second part was

the use of PLeG to teach and engage children in various subjects to reinforce what has been learned in school. In the third and final part, each group was involved in play group activities following an agenda built on the participants' needs.

The regular interactions between the educators, project team, and the children made it possible to create a file for each child focused on their needs and strengths. This helped to tailor the HH program and to identify children who needed special attention. At school, it was not possible to assess or address the specific needs of children due to the large number of children and the teaching method. In the HH program, we discovered children in the primary grades who had very poor verbal and writing skills or were illiterate. There were also children like Jas (whose story we are going to tell you soon) who exhibited bigger struggles. In order to meet these children's needs, the second part of the HH program offered more specific activities in smaller groups of children. We identified a growing number of children who needed specific care; however, the project had no increase in human resources; therefore, we introduced shifts and limited children's attendance to HH every second day. This was a hard decision and difficult to manage, but it helped to provide more care to the most troubled children with great benefits, especially for those in kindergarten and elementary grades. Moreover, the smaller groups helped to create a stronger and more positive relationship between educators and children.

Project specifics: "developing play together" with teachers

The teachers were selected by the school board and participated on an average of two experiential training days every three months. Informed by the field visits, each training focused on different psychoeducation topics and skills development, with the purpose of regularly including new modalities in the school interactions. The project was organised to exert a positive impact on three levels:

1 *Children* benefited from extended and effective learning opportunities.
2 *Teachers* increased their competence and satisfaction in their work.
3 *Schools* could count on highly regarded skilled professionals who could provide extra support for the other teachers and children's parents.

Training component

All teachers we worked with were extremely playful and showed great adaptation capacities as they engaged in different approaches during the long training days. Nevertheless, we had to consider that most of them, like their own students, grew up in an environment full of challenges and were trained with the same strict discipline and didactic academic rote "hurried style". Some of them had lived through the horror of the war or the harshness of it through their parents. Considering the critical socio-economic conditions in the region 20 and 40 years before, it is highly likely that their living conditions offered few learning opportunities and occasions to engage in their own pretend play.

The experience of working with people from different cultural contexts taught us that a precious component of our work is to be aware that what we teach is not always relevant to the participants (especially at the beginning). The training is not immediately absorbed and integrated. People do not immediately grasp the relevance of how the training could meet the needs of their context. In recognition that the training demands a great adaptation for the participants, we applied the following principles:

1   Teach using the PLeG model, make the learning for teachers active and motivating, and provide practical examples of attitude, activities, and abilities that could be applied with their own students.
2   Apply culturally respectful adaptations to the different abilities and provide opportunities to discuss the reasons for why we suggested the changes (with the support of the neuroscience).
3   Consider three phases in the training process: a pre-training assessment with the formulation of the training objectives, the actual training days, and the post-training assistance in classes (group supervision and individual coaching).

From our perspective, the implementation of these three points set the foundation for "good practice" (see Chapter 1), increasing the possibilities to amplify the dimensions of respect, effectiveness, and safety within the project (Mochi, forthcoming 2022).

The entire program included a large psychoeducational component aimed at supporting the application of different play activities and relational skills in the daily class interactions. The initial stage focused on introducing recreational play activities starting with one activity per day and then adding play rituals to the daily routine. Then play-based activity was introduced to manage the engagement level of children. In a second stage, teachers learnt how to apply Child-Centred Play Therapy skills (VanFleet et al., 2010) during episodes of free play with the idea to generalise these skills in the daily class routine. In later stages, teachers learnt how to use play activities to promote self-regulation and to stimulate children's active participation in learning.

A big component of the training started to focus on the importance of developing pretend play abilities by studying the Learn to Play Therapy approach and its application in the school context. The application of LtP in the classroom requires specific skills and a lot of competences starting from the "knowledge of the development of pretend play across 6 key play skills" (Stagnitti, 2021: 51). The previous experience in practising child-centred abilities helped teachers to acquire some of the skills such as attuning to the child, describing the play as the child played, and joining the child in role-play (op. cit.: 51–52). The other eight skills required a lot of effort and practice. LtP group approach implies the ability to identify the developmental level of pretend play per each group age, prepare suitable activities and play materials accordingly, identify those children who need extra support, and develop the ability to engage them. Not an easy task in any context and especially when pretend play was new to the educators who had not had opportunities in their own lives to pretend in play. Nevertheless, we were confident that the relationship built with the educators during the long playful weekends would help us to work together to add this new pillar to the project.

Following some of the LtP principles, we organised training making it enjoyable, understandable, engaging, and offering many opportunities to practice with variations (op. cit.). In some of the training, we divided the teachers into small groups and each group would focus on one ability, for instance, "object substitutions", and play all the scenarios for each of the six developmental levels of the ability. Another scenario was to play all the six abilities for the same stage of development simultaneously. There was discussion from each group as they practised the skills. We also introduced LtP role-play sessions where teachers were involved in using one, two, or all the skills with children showing different levels of pretend play abilities. In order to extend the experience and pleasure in this sort of play, we introduced narrative activities in which different groups had to create a story based on one or more prompts, given sentences, or scenarios. Similar activities were also performed using dramatisation instead of narrative. Pretend play was practised from different angles and all teachers showed great playfulness.

After almost two years, playing in class with children became natural and children were no longer overwhelmed when exposed to toys. Compared to the other project's activities, this component required extra commitment for the teachers, but they immediately incorporated the new approach in the free time starting with the assessment of the play ability level of children and adapting the setting and the play materials. They also learnt how to identify children who needed more support. The phase that needed more practice was the skill of engaging children who struggled the most. For these children, extra support was given by our team using a lot of demonstrations, shared work, and supervision. The expat team visited twice every three months, but the local team could focus on more vulnerable children twice per month. Teachers working with younger children or children who had more difficulties received longer visits and pretend play thrived in all the classes involved.

With teachers working with older children, the team was occupied with creating adjustments to the setting and guaranteeing the availability of play and creative material. We observed play sessions, sometimes we played near the teacher to model some abilities, and we interacted with children who had more challenges. We always left the class management to the teacher. My (Claudio) impression was extremely positive as the level of enjoyment of the teachers, and their ability in using the PLeG method became increasingly capable and natural.

Program-specific: "developing play together" with children

Children welcomed the play novelties with enthusiasm only as they can do. It was a big change for them when teachers started to introduce play activities in the school setting. The use of bamboo and sticks by the teachers against the students was gradually replaced by different moments of play that helped to create a safer and more inviting atmosphere during the long curricular days. Children became more active and interested in learning. Meanwhile, teachers could use their playfulness and play-based repertoire to manage different and difficult moments. From the early stages of the project, the "Talking ball game" became one of the most used activities to invite children to talk and participate. Like magic, the feared moment of being called by the teacher became a playful interaction each child wanted to be part of. The game started very simply: "When you receive the ball, you say 'thank you (name)', then you say the name of somebody else and you throw the ball to him/her". The teachers used all possible variations of this activity, but the simple use of the ball added a spark of movement and involved regulation skills such as inhibition and working memory (Barkley, 1997). It created a new dimension in the class dynamics. From this start, teachers were supported in gradually inserting play activities to help children to regulate their level of activity, inviting them to join traditional games or using other games like "Simon says". According to the children's regulation needs, the sentence "Simon says dance or jump!" would be alternated with "Simon says breath" or "move slowly or extra slowly". The ingredients of play and sense of competence worked for everybody.

For children, in particular, the progressive introduction of different play activities and relational abilities of the teachers increased their active engagement, learning, and pleasure in experiencing a different relationship with teachers. Along with this, a turning point for children was the introduction of the free play time and the appearance of toys in the classrooms. Many young children had never seen a toy before and they could not refrain from grabbing them or putting them into their bags. For the younger children, the first play episodes ended in a big fight over toys. Most of the sessions were spent in restoring calm and peace among children. It was quite a process to reach the point when children could choose quietly which toys to play with within class. Initially, the youngest were given objects and were invited to play sitting at their desks. For the older, we found the "weird walk" (Stagnitti, 2021: 161) extremely useful. In order to get to the toys, teachers prompted children to dramatise different kinds of walking: turtle, old man, tired and older turtle, and so on. When the noise was too loud, moving like a fish worked very well to restore silence. Time and teachers' modelling helped to make this activity more fun and the beginning of play time smoother.

From playing at the desk, the children's play gradually moved to more space within the class but, as described before, children's level of play did not improve. The moment we understood that children needed support to be able to play, the whole process became much easier as we added in LtP. Teachers were studying and developing their own LtP skills, and our team supported the classes. Children loved to see different ways to play; they enjoyed observing and imitating the adults. Their extreme curiosity made the process of engagement very easy and gradually many children could initiate their own play.

For the vast majority of children, the poverty of imaginary play skills was caused by the lack of a stimulating environment. After one week of introducing pretend play activities, we observed many children initiating their own pretend play. This allowed our team to focus on those who needed more attention. Older children were curious and very responsive. To increase play abilities and sustain the engagement of the children, we spent more time in setting up and preparing and also creating new material. For example, we included thematic corners in the classroom such as playing market, police, hairdresser, or school. Alternatively, children could plan and prepare their own play scene or set it up for others based on ideas from their school topics. The children's engagement in pretend play, plus the PLeG method, created a positive circle of learning with academic studies that provided stimulation for play and more complex play that expanded children's creative interaction during the lesson.

Case study

I don't know exactly his age, as few children are registered at birth, but Jas is an adolescent now. He is attending a Technical School, and he is happy with this new adventure. He no longer attends the HH centre, but he visits it often when he comes back home. He likes to see friends and spend time in the places of his childhood.

The first time I saw him was five years before, during a play activity I was leading. Over time I noticed he liked the motor activity and did not engage in any other play. At school, he could imitate other children by answering the teacher's questions in the group. In the big and noisy class, he was able to give the impression he had knowledge (which he did not have). He did not speak on his own. He was extremely quiet, often punished, and constantly in charge of different school chores.

Reading his file, I understood that his story was of severe early neglect. After a few years, his grandmother took him with her. His family was one of the most needy among those supported by the SOS Distant Adoption Project. Jas was extremely rigid physically and a great observer. I could never figure out entirely Jas's difficulties, but for the fact, he was struggling with learning. I heard his voice in class and his shouting during football, but otherwise he did not communicate verbally and, even though he was probably around 8 years, he was basically illiterate.

During one of my visits to the school, something captured my attention in a classroom: four of Jas's classmates were restraining him and the teacher was beating him with a stick. The reason was that he did not answer some questions during the lesson. The teacher believed Jas was a stubborn child, but he did not realise Jas did not know the answers. In class, Jas tried to be invisible by hiding behind the crowd of classmates, the noise, and the collective repetitions of rote learning. The teacher was not angry at Jas, in fact, when I interrupted the teacher, he was surprised and explained that he was imparting discipline to help Jas. I can't forget the scene with Jas crying silently, the children restraining him with nervous giggles, and everything looking absurd and normal at the same time. It was painful to think that this was the everyday reality for some children; hiding in fear, then getting caught, ashamed, and hurt. From that moment, my relationship with Jas changed. I soon noticed he was curious about our team and what we proposed, but we had a busy agenda as we set up the foundations for the project and, as mentioned, he was able to stay invisible. While other children were very communicative and interactive, Jas was overwhelmed by them.

Play story – starting a career

Jas was a regular participant at the HH centre from a young age and his school was the nearest to our office and house in Southern Nigeria. During free play in the HH program, when he could not join older children in the playground, he was passive. He followed other children's play, but he did not seem to know what to do and how to join them. In a project that involved so many children and limited space and resources, it took time before we could start providing more specific attention to children who needed specific care. It also took time to realise that, apart from football where he was joyfully engaged running up and down the field, Jas could not play. Introducing him to a smaller group of children was a big change for him. On these occasions, during free time he discovered puzzles and his afternoon time changed completely as he engaged in a different type of play.

We started to introduce Learn to Play Therapy. This was an additional step in his "career as a player" when we reduced the number of toys and started to show him how to use the toys in pretend play. He still played with puzzles, but now he could think about other ways to play. He discovered trucks and cars and finally started to move from the table. It was beautiful to see him playing moving the toys all around the room, but for him, there were too many distractions and he needed another person to help him keep focused on the play. He was not yet involved in other children's play nor responding to the play alternatives we were proposing.

Jas needed to see and practice different play abilities at his own pace. He needed a one-to-one intervention. In individual sessions, he needed to be engaged to see that the truck could move, make a lot of noise, and you could also load a certain amount of blocks in the truck. He needed to see that the loads of blocks could then be tipped out and organised. I remember when he noticed that different vehicles could be used in similar play scenarios and the dolls could organise the blocks. When the doll started to be involved in constructions, a moment of change in his play was marked. He laughed heartily, and his joint attention became "imitation with understanding" (Stagnitti,

2021). From that moment, it was a brief step for Jas to begin to initiate his own play. When it came to building, he no longer imitated me; instead, his doll had her own ideas about the kind of dwelling she wanted to build and had her preferences for what material to use.

LtP is very powerful. When I saw this silent child imposing his ideas and developing his narrative, I was happy but also tempted to add some enriching elements to his play. LtP requires a constant balance between following the child's initiative and facilitating new abilities by challenging the child to a more complex level of play. I learnt this balance by using the attunement and description abilities when Jas was developing his play, and then proposing alternatives using another doll just when he needed support. For example, my doll was getting tired easily and needed to rest and eat. He liked the idea of other characters driving the truck and having a life. As humans do, these characters followed a hierarchy of needs, so once they satisfied their basic needs they started to commit to more refined ones: a nicer house, work, a hobby, animals to take care of, different varieties of food to buy, and so on. LtP one-to-one requires greater preparation in "developing goals" and in "understanding when to engage the client", and I admit it was a steep learning curve. He was confident and engaged, but I was also conscious that I could confuse him if I proposed something too complicated in the play. Reviewing his PPE-DC was a great support, and I could see clearly he was struggling with play scripts and object substitution abilities and was not flexible with new ideas. I concentrated on these play skills, and eventually, the dress-up clothing became alive and the doctor's gown was not just something to wear but facilitated ideas for a new play script that supported a specific role in play. In object substitution, a box became an additional means to transport the construction material. Jas was becoming more flexible in his play.

Learn to Play Therapy would have been ideal for Jas from the beginning, but this was not possible given the situation. When I was absent, he was part of Learn to Play groups and could continue what we started to practice in individual sessions. At the time, our local team was not yet trained to the point where they could work individually with children. The project had several limitations but also valid points. We could observe children while they had the opportunity to experience similar activities both at school and in the HH centre. During the short sessions, we had every second day I could also observe Jas. Over time, I noticed that he started to be active in groups and it is in a group that I heard him talking. In the Learn to Play group, he preferred his own play but started to observe others and exchange toys with them. It was parallel play but still a great improvement.

In my absence, the group work was highly beneficial for him. He started to use puppets in interactions with other children. He was in the class with younger children, but he was enjoying it. Our second cycle of intense individual sessions was shorter. We did four more individual sessions where I mostly followed his initiatives in play. I did introduce variations to the play actions and added some complexity where this was needed.

Jas did 11 individual sessions but a great number of small and bigger group play. In the last group I co-facilitated, he was playing "police and thieves" with others. The play included fighting, chasing, arresting, jail, and judgment. He was very energetic but also well regulated. I remember he was really enjoying the play. He was communicating openly with other players, negotiating the details of scripts when needed. For his age, he was still behind but totally engrossed in his play and interactive in all other activities. Every day he was picking up something new, and I could see multi-faceted improvements.

Jas's story is unique, but it has common elements with other children we worked with. I choose to tell his play story because his case represents an application of LtP that combined individual and group play and also because of the recollection of that invisible link we created when I took his side during his punishment. This made him even more special to me. In addition, his progression in play and learning mirrored the improvement and the refinement in the project. We began our project with less specialised activities, and as we progressed, we tailored the intervention using more specific and suitable methodologies to meet the needs of the population, building capacity of educators so that we became unnecessary.

Conclusion

The overall experience offered human and professional food for thought, observable positive outcomes, and limitations. The project did not have a research focus, which could have been an added value for further crisis interventions. Over five years, we collected much data through field observations, videos, supervision files from teachers' practice, and files on children attending HH. Collecting these data was planned from the beginning, so we could adjust the project, offer relevant and suitable training, and provide evidence for "good practice". On the other hand, a research component could have supported the project by providing empirical evidence on the outcomes, the writing of scientific publications, and increased chances to get financial support from diversified sources. However, considering the number of teachers and children, adding the research component would have meant allocation of human resources exclusively to research, which was not possible at that time.

In retrospect, from the second year of the project, the number of local and foreign human resources should have been increased. The number of public and private schools involved in the project increased gradually over the five years as well as the number of children frequenting HH. The project gave us insight into how to use LtP in such a project, and the positive outcomes increased our credibility and connections in the whole region. In the fifth year, a new three-year project was formulated. The proposal included working with local universities that trained teachers. We had the full support of the Ministry of Education and, considering the precious experience we built, we wanted to reach as many professionals as possible and as soon as possible in their education training. Despite this, the project budget did not allow for expansion.

Last but not least, the conditions of political and economic instability in the country and the level of generalised violence in the region increased dramatically. It became dangerous to travel to the various schools. Military roadblocks were frequent and unpredictable, and recruiting professionals from abroad was equally difficult. When the five-year project ended, the new one could not start.

On the one hand, the positive impact of the project can be analysed by considering the changes in the complexity of the children's play. First, the "story of Onyochi" is an example of changes in play ability. Onyochi was a big doll stocked in HH, which had been neglected for many years. When free play was introduced, Onyochi started going around on children's shoulders, but she was soon dropped somewhere. Over time, she became "alive" (this is the ability to decentre from self, Stagnitti, 2021), and children started to feed and take care of her. After a few more months, we noticed that Onyochi's activities became more complex: she had a friend to play with, she went to the hairdresser, to buy food, she moved around by car, and she went to school to learn and sometimes also to teach.

Onyochi is a simple but great story of play development, and it is our belief that the project touched the community in different ways. Teachers were playfully engaged with children; they brought different expressive materials and used toys to involve children during class. Our colleague Isabella says that one of the characteristics of the effectiveness of a project is that the local colleagues are capable to carry on without us because their training has given them a "new reality". This reflects Vygotsky's perspective (1978: 57) as new abilities exist initially as external activities and only after a series of developmental events, the interpersonal process becomes internalised and the new abilities can be self-directed and even mastered.

Two relevant long-term results have occurred. First, the educators responsible for HH reached a level of ability and skills in managing different methodologies, including "Learn to Play approach in schools", and are providing encompassing and enriching experiences to hundreds of children daily. Second, during the last visit to HH's kindergarten, we noticed very young children, after their first month of attendance, exhibiting their own self-initiated pretend play. In little time, their play was more advanced than the older children in the previous years, and the best part is that they learnt from an enriched environment of peers and play resources.

Our last visit was extremely encouraging for two reasons: children learnt by watching and interacting with more competent children. For example, they were observing everything Onyochi could do and, in general, they were being exposed to a more stimulating environment compared to all the other children before them. The other good news was that following the HH program, children were becoming more competent with skilled adults ready to recognise and follow their lead. The benefits of the project continue.

References

Andronico, M.P. and Guerney, B. (1967) 'The potential application of filial therapy to the school situation', *Journal of School Psychology*, 6(1), 2–7, Doi: 10.1016/0022–4405(67)90057-X.

Axline, V. (1974) *Play therapy*, New York, NY: Ballantine Books.

Barkley, R. (1997) *ADHD and the nature of self control*, New York, NY: Guilford Press.

Bodrova, E., Germeroth, C. and Leong, D.J. (2013) 'Play and self-regulation. Lessons from Vygotsky', *American Journal of Play*, 6, 111–123.

Bodrova, E. and Leong, D.J. (2006) *Tools of the mind*, Melbourne: Pearson Australia Pty Limited.

Brooks, R. (2009) *The play of children: Lessening stress and increasing self-control*, available: www.drrobertbrooks.com/wp2/wp-content/uploads/2009/10/The-Play-of-Children-Lessening-Stress-and-Increasing-Self-Control.pdf [accessed 22 July 2021].

Creaghe, N., Quinn, S. and Kidd, E. (2021) 'Symbolic play provides a fertile context for language development', *Infancy*, 26(6), 980–1010, Doi: 10.1111/infa.12422.

Dabiri Golchin, M., Mirzakhani, M., Stagnitti, K. Dabiri Golchin, M. and Mehdi, R. (2017) 'Psychometric properties of Persian version of child-initiated pretend play assessment for Iranian children', *Iran Journal of Pediatrics*, 27, e7053, Doi: 10.5812/ijp.7053.

Davidson, D. and Stagnitti, K. (2021) 'The process of learn to play therapy with parent-child dyads with children who have autism spectrum disorder', *Australian Occupational Therapy Journal*, 68, 419–433, Doi: 10.1111/1440–1630.12751.

de Haan, D., Vriens-van Hoogdalem, A-G., Zeijlmans, K. and Boom, J. (2021) 'Metacommunication in social pretend play: two dimensions', *International Journal of Early Years Education*, 29, 405–419, Doi: 10.1080/09669760.2020.1778451.

Dender, A. and Stagnitti, K. (2011) 'The development of the Indigenous child initiated pretend play assessment: selection of play materials and administration', *Australian Occupational Therapy Journal*, 58, 34–42, Doi: 10.1111/j.1440–1630.2010.00905.x.

Dender, A. and Stagnitti, K. (2017) 'Content and cultural validity in the development of the Indigenous play partner scale', *Australian Occupational Therapy Journal*, 64, 283–293, Doi: 10.1111/1440–1630.12355.

Drewes, A.A. (2001) 'The possibilities and challenges in using play therapy in schools', in C.E., Schaefer, L.J., Carey and A.A., Drewes (eds.) *School-based play therapy*, Hoboken, New Jersey: John Wiley & Sons Inc., 41–61.

Dunst, C.J., Hamby, D., Trivette, C.M., Raab, M. and Bruder, M.B. (2000) 'Everyday family and community life and children's naturally occurring learning opportunities', *Journal of Early intervention*, 23(3), 151–164.

Eberle, S. (2014) 'The elements of play. Toward a philosophy and a definition of play', *American Journal of Play*, 6, 214–233, available: www.journalofplay.org/sites/www.journalofplay.org/files/pdf-articles/6-2-article-elements-of-play.pdf [accessed 16 September 2021].

Elkind, D. (1987) *Miseducation: preschoolers at risk*, New York, NY: Alfred A Knopf, Inc.

Garbarino, J. (1998) *Supporting parents in a socially toxic environment*, available: https://parenthood.library.wisc.edu/Garbarino/Garbarino.html [accessed 11 August 2021].

Garbarino, J. (1999) *Educating children in a socially toxic environment*, available: www.theforum journal.org/1999/12/04/educating-children-in-a-socially-toxic-environment/ [accessed 19 July 2021].

Ginsburg, K.R. (2007) 'The importance of play in promoting healthy child development and maintaining strong parent-child bonds', *Pediatrics*, 119(1), 182–191.

Gosso, Y., De Lima Salum e Morais, M. and Otta, E. (2007) 'Pretend play of Brazilian children: A window into different cultural worlds', *Journal of Cross-Cultural Psychology*, 38, 539–558, Doi: 10.1177/0022022107305237.

Guerney, B., Jr. (1964) 'Filial therapy: Description and rationale', *Journal of Consulting Psychology*, 28(4), 304–310.

Haight, W.L., Wang, X-l, Fung, H.H., Williams, K. and Mintz, J. (1999) 'Universal, developmental, and variable aspects of young children's play: A cross-cultural comparison of pretending at home', *Child Development*, 70, 1477–1488.

Hirsh-Pasek, K. and Michnick Golinkoff, R. (2020) 'Playful learning and raising successful children in the twenty-first century: An interview with Kathy Hirsh-Pasek and Roberta Mmichnick Golinkoff', *American Journal of Play*, 13, 1–20, available: www.journalofplay. org/sites/www.journalofplay.org/files/pdf-articles/13-1-Article-1-Playful-Learning.pdf [accessed 3 June 2021].

Inter-Agency Standing Committee and the European Commission (2021) *INFORM Risk Index 2022*, Document released 31 August 2021 by the European Commission Joint Research Centre, available: https://drmkc.jrc.ec.europa.eu/inform-index [accessed 4 January 2022].

Lee, Y.C., Chan, P-C., Lin, S-K., Chen, C-T., Huang, C-Y. and Chen, K-L. (2016) 'Correlation patterns between pretend play and playfulness in children with autism spectrum disorder, developmental delay, and typical development', *Research in Autism Spectrum Disorders*, 24, 29–38, Doi: 10.1016/J.RASD.2016.01.006.

Lucisano, R.V., Pfeifer, L.I., Santos, J.L.F. and Stagnitti, K. (2020) 'Construct validity of the child-initiated pretend play assessment for 3 year old Brazilian children', *Australian Occupational Therapy Journal*, 68, 43–53, Doi: 10.1111/1440–1630.12697.

Masten, A.S. (2009) 'Ordinary magic: Lessons from research on resilience in human development', *Education Canada*, 49(3), 28–32.

Mochi, C. (forthcoming 2022) *Beyond the clouds: An autoethnographic research exploring the good practice in crisis settings*, Ann Arbor, MI: Loving Healing Press.

Morrison, M. and Pretz Helker, W. (2010) 'Child-teacher relationship training using the power of the child – teacher relationship as a school-based mental health intervention', in A.A., Drewes and C.E., Schaefer (eds.) *School based play therapy*, 2nd edn., Hoboken, NJ: Wiley, 181–196.

Nicolopoulou, A., Barbosa de Sa, A., Ilgaz, H. and Brockmeyer, C. (2010) 'Using the transformative power of play to educate hearts and minds: from Vygotsky to Vivian Paley and beyond', *Mind, Culture, and Activity*, 17, 42–58.

O'Connor, C. and Stagnitti, K. (2011) 'Play, behaviour, language and social skills: The comparison of a play and a non-play intervention within a specialist school setting', *Research in Developmental Disabilities*, 32, 1205–1211, Doi: 10.1016/j.ridd.2010.12.037.

Panksepp, J. (2010) 'Science of the brain as a gateway to understanding play', *American Journal of Play*, 2, 245–277.

Peabody, M.A., Johnson, D. and Hightower, A.D. (2010) 'Primary project: An evidence-based approach', in A.A., Drewes and C.E., Schaefer (eds.) *School based play therapy*, 2nd edn., Hoboken, NJ: Wiley, 163–180.

Perry, B.D., Pollard, R., Blakely, T., Baker, W. and Vigilante, D. (1995) *Childhood trauma, the neurobiology of adaptation and 'use-dependent' development of the brain: How 'states' become 'traits'*, available: www.childtrauma.org/ctamaterials/states_traits.asp [accessed 13 March 2021].

Post, P. (2001) 'Child-centered play therapy for at-risk elementary school children', in C.E., Schaefer, L.J., Carey and A.A., Drewes (eds.) *School-based play therapy*, Hoboken, NJ: Wiley, 105–122.

Rakoczy, H. (2008a) 'Taking fiction seriously: children understand the normative structure of joint pretence games', *Developmental Psychology*, 44, 1195–1201, Doi: 10.1037/0012–1649.44.4.1195.

Rakoczy, H. (2008b) 'Pretence as individual and collective intentionality', *Mind & Language*, 23, 499–517, Doi: 10.1111/j.1468–0017.2008.00357.

Reddy, L.A. (2010) 'Group play interventions for children with attention deficit/hyperactivity disorder', in A.A., Drewes and C.E., Schaefer (eds.) *School based play therapy*, 2nd edn., Hoboken, NJ: Wiley, 307–329.

Reynolds, E., Stagnitti, K. and Kidd, E. (2011) 'Play, language and social skills of children aged 4–6 years attending a play based curriculum school and a traditionally structured classroom curriculum school in low socio-economic areas', *Australian Journal of Early Childhood*, 36(4), 120–130.

Richard, S., Baud-Bovy, G., Clerc-Georgy, A. and Gentaz, E. (2021) 'The effects of a "pretend play-based training" designed to promote the development of emotion comprehension, emotion regulation, and pro-social behaviour in 5- to 6-year-old Swiss children', *British Journal of Psychology*, 112, 690–719, Doi: 10.1111/bjop.12484.

Sameroff, A.J., Seifer, R., Barocas, R., Zax, M. and Greenspan, S. (1987) 'Intelligence quotient scores of 4-year-old children: social-environmental risk factors', *Pediatrics*, 79(3), 343–50, PMID: 3822634.

Shore, R. (1997) *Rethinking the brain*, New York, NY: Families and Work Institute.

SOSolidarietà and INA International Academy for Play Therapy Studies and Psychosocial Projects (2012) *Progetto Crescere Insieme*, internal document.

Stagnitti, K. (2010) 'Helping preschool and kindergarten teachers foster play in the classroom', in A.A., Drewes and C.E., Schaefer (eds.) *School based play therapy*, 2nd edn., Hoboken, NY: Wiley, 145–161.

Stagnitti, K. (2017) *Pretend play enjoyment developmental checklist: Manual*, Melbourne: Learn to Play.

Stagnitti, K. (2021) *Learn to play therapy. Principles, process, and practical activities*, Melbourne: Learn to Play.

Stagnitti, K., Bailey, A., Hudspbeth-Stevenson, E., Reynolds, R. and Kidd, E. (2016) 'An investigation into the effect of play-based instruction on the development of play skills and oral language: A 6-month longitudinal study', *Journal of Early Childhood Research*, 14(4), 389–406, Doi: 10.1177/1476718X15579741.

Stagnitti, K. and Lewis, F.M. (2015) 'The importance of the quality of preschool children's pretend play ability to the subsequent development of semantic organisation and narrative re-telling skills in early primary school', *International Journal of Speech-Language Pathology*, 17(2), 148–158.

Tigerstied, H. and Stagnitti, K. (2014) 'The ChIPPA in Finland', paper presentation, *European Sensory Integration Congress*, Naantali, Finland.

UNDP United Nations Development Programme (2019) 'The next frontier: human development and the anthropocene. briefing note for countries on the 2020 human development', available: http://hdr.undp.org/sites/default/files/Country-Profiles/NGA.pdf [accessed 2 December 2021].

VanFleet, R. and Guerney, L. (eds.) (2003) *Casebook of filial therapy*, Boiling Springs, PA: Play Therapy Press.

VanFleet, R., Sywulak, A.E. and Sniscak, C.C. (eds.) (2010) *Child-centered play therapy*, New York, NY: The Guilford Press.

Vygotsky, L. (2016) 'Play and its role in the mental development of the child', *International Research in Early Childhood Education*, 7(2), 3–25, available: https://files.eric.ed.gov/fulltext/EJ1138861.pdf.

Vygotsky, L.S. (1978) *Mind in society: Development of higher psychological processes*, Cambridge, MA: Harvard University Press.

Wadley, C. and Stagnitti, K. (2020) 'The experiences of school staff in the implementation of a learn to play programme', *International Journal of Early Years Education*, 1–14, Doi: 10.1080/09669760.2020.1848526.

Whitebread, D. and O'Sullivan, L. (2012) 'Preschool children's social pretend play: Supporting the development of metacommunication, metacognition and self-regulation', *International Journal of Play*, 1, 197–213.

Zosh, J.M., Hirsh-Pasek, K., Hopkins, E.J., Jensen, H., Liu, C., Neale, D., Solis, L. and Whitebread, D. (2018) 'Accessing the inaccessible: Redefining play as a spectrum', *Frontiers in Psychology*, 9, 1–12. Doi: 10.3389/fpsyg.2018.01124.

6 Nature-based Play Therapy interventions in the digital age

Maggie Fearn

The theoretical framework draws on the author's clinical practice and a synthesis of theory from human development, applied neurobiology, somatics, and psychodynamic theory and focuses on the role of nature as a therapeutic ally for the play therapist and child in the process of regulating and nourishing a child's sense of where they are, who they are, and what being safe feels like. The case study vignettes show that immersive play experiences in the natural environment promote a child's growth, development, and healing, and evoke the possibilities, wonder, and limits of being a human being.

Suzanne Simard (2013) describes the complex inter-relationships between trees and other life forms in forests and woodlands. She was one of the first to scientifically prove that all plant life in the undisturbed forest is interconnected underground via a vast network of communication pathways provided by mycorrhizal fungi associations. The fungi filaments provide a lattice of communication channels where two-way messages flow via chemical and ionic interconnections. These networks bear more than a metaphoric resemblance to the human endocrine and nervous systems. What is more, Simard identifies how the oldest trees in the forest provide nourishment and support for thousands of mixed-species saplings, mothering their communities and all who live off them through these dynamic earth channels. Life in this sense is deeply interconnected, mutually beneficial, and communal. All species within a natural community cooperate with each other. Survival depends on being entangled with other species, belonging in relationship to each other and with those yet to be born, including all species who directly or indirectly live off and with the land, the air, and the water that flows through it.

I am seated at my computer in my clinic, surrounded by books and paper. Large windows let in light, sky, and the impression of constant movement and colour, bringing the surrounding woodland garden into my workspace. It is late October, and outside my office, the great Welsh oak is shedding. Each time the gusts of wind sway her branches a flock of ochre leaves flutter to the ground, animating the air with their spinning, floating fall. I leave my desk to run out and try to catch them. I am dazzled by the low sunlight and the mosaic of yellow, bronze, and ochre pieces already on the ground. The air is musky and warm and the wind snatches at my hair. The sun is nearer the horizon

DOI: 10.4324/9781003252375-7

at this time of year and casts its spell of light over us briefly. I am anticipating the winter with every cell of my body. I can because I too am entangled in this place, I have experienced 31 winters here. I have witnessed the mother tree prepare 31 times over her support for our community through the annual cycle. She was a sapling many generations before I was born, yet I feel viscerally connected to her and the community she has engendered that provides us with everything we need to survive. I know where I am here, I feel at home, this is where I belong. I explore outwards into the world from here, knowing I have a secure base, and when I return here, I feel safe.

The concept of a secure base is fundamental to attachment theory, and the infant's orientation in relation to their primary caregiver is profoundly spatial. Our first question is not "who am I?" it is "where am I?" (Straus, 1966). Our very first experience of relationship is environmental, and it is through movement and touch that we experience "being here" within the living body of our mother, who in turn exists and responds to the world through her senses in environmental relationship.

> *In utero*, in symbiotic relationship, the developing child has the capacity to resonate with, and move in relation to, the sound, vibrations and pulsations of their mother's heart rate, breathing pattern, emotions, voice and visceral movements, as well as the ability to detect changes in the mother's body position in space. The first environment of relationship is the living body of the mother: within this living environment, the nervous system of the baby develops and is imprinted with the primal neurological information that initially prefigures her unique way of perceiving and interacting with inner and outer worlds. *In utero* experiences establish patterns of interaction that develop, via the birth experience, into the post-natal attachment relationship.
>
> (Fearn and Troccoli, 2017: 104–105)

By the third trimester *in utero*, the mother's and foetus's senses are fully functioning in syncrony, informed by complex environmental interactions. After birth, the infant's nervous system responds and adapts to environmental information from the perspective of the primary attachment relationship. The newborn infant is entirely dependent on the relationship with her carer and their shared environment for survival, and development occurs through repeat experiences forming associative patterns between sensing, perceiving, feeling and responding, forming implicit memory, and informing consciousness. Throughout this formative period, the infant inhabits a universe of sensation, forming associations between implicit memory traces and first receptive, then productive language. These associations create meaning out of playing with the sensory perception of their environment. They make sense of experience in relationship with significant older, wiser, caring beings – human and other-than-human – in their lives. If the care the infant receives activates her ability to self-regulate her responses to environmental stimulation, and her nervous system maintains a tolerable range of arousal, the territory of her lived world will be for the most part developmentally satisfying, expansive, fascinating, and playful.

In secure attachment, early experiences of consistent relational attunement, in which the mother is invested in anticipating and responding to her infant's needs in a safe and supportive environment, are crucial in the first six months after birth (Winnicott, 1949; Stern, 1985). Communication occurs via pre-verbal, sensory, and embodied channels. It is a dance between nervous systems, the infant's immature responses modulated and regulated through rhythmic movement, prosody, and touch by her primary carer, who in turn is contained by the loving care of family and community, in an environment that provides and supports, in direct response to the care invested in it. The infant's developing sense of self is nurtured in community: perceiving *where* I am provides the ground for discovering *who* I am.

In times of stress, the human autonomic nervous system seeks out support from community and environment. Porges' polyvagal theory (1995, 2007) proposes that we have evolved to cope with threat by socially engaging with each other and learning how to be effective actors in our environment. This calms the sympathetic nervous system stress response sufficiently for us to be able to think through strategies for survival beyond the fight/flight reflex. Infants cannot self-regulate arousal states and, for better or worse, they are reliant on engagement with their primary carer at times of stress. This early experience matures into patterns of response to stress across the lifespan. Research into regulated stress response details how a normal autonomic nervous system response to threat (i.e. a temporary physiological state) has the opportunity to recover homeostasis in connection with a regulating other person or environment (Perry, 2001; Norwood et al., 2019). However, if a child lives in a chaotic, frightening environment, their autonomic nervous system will be in a permanent state of arousal to threat, and their physiological state can become a permanent trait (Perry et al., 1995; Anda et al., 2006). If support is not available, the body prepares for flight or fight, and many children who have experienced relational trauma rely on avoidance or aggression as their default stress responses. If a child is too small to fight back and trapped in a dynamic of powerlessness and fear, the parasympathetic nervous system response can activate the final and most primitive survival response of fainting or dissociation: an acceptance that nothing can change and a collapse of autonomic functioning that is potentially life threatening (Perry et al., 1995).

Porges (2007) proposes that in order to continuously inform the polyvagal survival response, the human nervous system subliminally scans our surroundings for safety via our senses, orienting us in three-dimensional space and also modulating feedback from our major organs. He calls this process "neuroception", a neural process that evaluates risk and modulates vagal output via higher brain structures. This brings awareness to autonomic sensing for safety as a vital tool in self-regulation. Porges' work has contributed significantly to our understanding of human responses to threat, and Perry et al.'s conceptualisation of an unregulated threat response provides a rationale for explaining the spectrum of traumatic response, from hypervigilance to dissociation, which we see in so many children referred to play therapy.

Exploring the concept of continuous subliminal sensing gives further insight into a child's experience of being in the world when feeling safe and not activated by an imminent threat. The French philosopher, Merleau-Ponty (2012/1945, translated 2012), distinguishes between two kinds of perception, defined as analytical and phenomenological consciousness. In his somatic unravelling of Merleau-Ponty's conceptualisations, Hanna (1970) associates analytical consciousness with the sympathetic nervous system. This suggests heightened arousal, focused attention, and a searching mode that is able to distinguish and highlight specific identifying information from a multi-sensory background. Edward Wilson (1984), entomologist and respected naturalist, explains that in a state of calm attention, the sympathetic nervous system makes us alert for the unexpected, able to assess possible risks and respond accordingly. This adaptation to the environment resonates with the concept of assimilation in child development (Piaget, 1977). The ability to assess and adapt to incoming information through sensing, perceiving, and action is vital for resilience and survival, and also for the vitality of engagement, which is typical of play: "being refreshed by the keen noses, sharp eyes and agile movements for the adaptational dance that we call life" (Hanna, 1970: 308).

Continuing his unravelling of Merleau-Ponty's conceptualisation of perception, Hanna associates phenomenological consciousness with the activation of the parasympathetic nervous system. The non-defensive parasympathetic mode is relaxed, diffuse, and accommodating. Phenomenological perception is open and curious about all incoming information, and senses meet stimuli without prior screening or discrimination. There is no effort expended on anticipating what something might mean, or intend. Everything just is. This mode of perception is a blissful immersive state, which allows for deep level learning, and re-patterning of the nervous system, resulting in fundamental developmental changes; a process Piaget (1977) refers to as accommodation.

Experiences in multi-sensory natural environments can induce both analytic and phenomenological perception, heightening our awareness of the human body as part of nature, not separate from it. In somatic thinking, the experience of being alive, i.e. "Me, the bodily being" is referred to as "soma" (Hanna, 1970: 35) and the awareness of complex felt senses of being alive, i.e. somatic intelligence, is referred to as the "bodymind" (Aposhyan, 2004) and "psyche-soma" (Winnicott, 1949). Children naturally embody the experience of being in the world as soma. In healthy development, both analytic and phenomenological consciousness are of equal survival and developmental value and are inherent in the regulatory patterns of early attachment relationships. Piaget (1977) refers to perceptual shifts between assimilation and accommodation in his conceptualisation of developmental growth. He considers children to be active participants in their own development, observing that their play behaviour is a reflection of how they think and express their embodied perceptions of reality from early infancy to adolescence. Landreth (2012) agrees that play activity is the child's preferred language of expression and therefore provides the optimum medium for child therapy. Czsikszentmihalyi (1990) explores the relationship between flow, creativity, and play, and Laevers (1993) associates immersion in play with deep level learning. Research into defining children's perceptions of play identifies that from a child's perspective, it is a profoundly felt embodied experience:

> Play to me is like my heart it beats and adds rhythmic beat to my life. I love playing all kinds of stuff because it makes me feel like things are happening in my head and everything I hear and see it makes me like life. Because of this feeling I feel good about myself. That's what play is to me.
>
> (11 Million, 2008: 16)

In an environment that provides support and nurture for the mother–infant dyad, they will together experience the flow between modalities of perception in a playful somatic relationship. If an infant has ongoing lived experience of being seen, heard, and loved and if her environment provides the support she needs at times of stress, then as she begins to explore, most of the time she will be reassured by familiar surroundings and able to become immersed in her local environs, investigate, and play independently and creatively with others and the unexpected things she finds. If something alerts her as a threat and she becomes alarmed she will stop playing and move to seek protection and reassurance from her caregiver's touch, voice, and particular energetic rhythm. This circular rhythmic process matures into the child's ability to reassure and regulate herself, drawing on inner resources in times of mild stress, and to seek support when feeling overwhelmed.

Early attachment experiences provide the blueprint from which a child creates expectations about relationships (Schore, 2001). Mild stress that results from momentary mis-attunement followed by reconnection is beneficial to developing a sense of the difference between self and other and is integral to the "good enough' attachment relationship. A felt sense of secure relationship is the foundation of the child's sense of self and is the first play environment, providing a sensation of "going on being", a core belief in the coherence and consistency of existence between inner and outer worlds that allows the child to trust in her self, her significant others, and her experiences in and of the world "out there" beyond the motility of the boundary of self (Winnicott, 1949).

An infant grounded in a nurturing environment has the best possible foundation for Hanna's "adaptational dance" into the world as a child (1970: 308). Children form their felt sense of reality through exploration and play that is intrinsically motivated and directed by the child's imagination in response to a contiguous stream of sensory information from both internal and external worlds. In free play, the young child is actively moving in the world, constantly processing sensory information, and making meaning and sense out of the spontaneous experience: always in dynamic relationship with the qualities, presences, and materials offered by their environment. Immersed in play in safe, contained natural settings, the flow from inner to outer worlds and back again encounters a little impediment, activating the child's congruency and authentic self-expression in response to perception. Stern (2010) identifies that a close match between kinaesthetic proprioceptive feedback and the stream of sensory information is essential, engendering self-awareness about how the body moves and where the body is located in each moment. Sensation and perception are the source of imagination, autonomy, and agency. The child expands her territorial knowledge and extends her "sensuous geography" (Rodaway, 1994) through play in a subjective flow from inner to outer world in which both the child and the environment are altered by the experience. This is the foundation of self/place relationship – each is essential to the other. For a child, being in the world is a continuous embodied experience. Whether situated in an urban or rural environment, indoors or outside, the playing child is deeply engaged physiologically through movement and touch in the processes of place-making, being, becoming, and developing emotional attachment with their community, both human and more-than-human.

Considering the environment as a significant presence and influence in attachment formation and child development contextualises and grounds the mother/infant dyad in a sense of place. It suggests a theoretical underpinning for considering the environmental context for all attachment histories and introduces the possibility of nature as nurturer in the attachment story. Being curious about the environmental context when considering families referred for therapeutic support may highlight the quality of environmental nurture available to both mother and infant in the early years, offering useful insight into the lived felt sense experiences of the mother–infant dyad during their formative time together.

Winnicott (1991) draws explicit parallels between the concept of original "good enough" mothering, and his conceptualisation of therapeutic relationship between the therapist and the child. His thinking about play is helpful in articulating the play therapist's motivation and clinical decision making inherent in working therapeutically with children. He visualises mother/infant play as both psychological and somatic territory: a space and time in which the child's unique inner sensory and perceptive experience can be expressed outwards without being immediately disavowed by reality. The mother's presence and attunement in effect keep objective reality at bay long enough for the child to experience efficacy. At first, the mother is invested totally in accommodating the baby's subjective reality (i.e. predominantly phenomenological perception), but over time, as the baby's resilience develops and the mother becomes less consistently available, the child will experience and will need to learn to tolerate disavowal of his omnipotence. Incidentally, Schore (2001) describes these felt sense moments of mis-attunement, and adjustment (i.e. assimilation) as evidence of the function of shame in healthy child development.

It is helpful to highlight here that play and development are inextricably linked, and that the nervous system, and therefore a child's play, is patterned by experience and develops sequentially. The impact of trauma depends on the timing of when the trauma occurred, and we can not only gain insight into a child's experience of trauma through observing their play but also provide developmentally appropriate reparative experiences utilising the inherent therapeutic powers of play (Schaefer and Drewes, 2014), therefore revisiting developmental stages of development and play in therapeutic relationship. In play therapy, children will seek out the kind of play they are hungry for. Jennings' (1999) developmental model of play therapy tracks the sequential model of therapeutics onto a developmental paradigm of play: broadly categorised as embodied play (sensorimotor play), projective play (symbolic play), and role-play (pretend play). This provides the play therapist with a developmental framework for understanding what the child is communicating about their developmental story through their choice of play (Prendiville, 2021). The proposal that the nervous system continues to respond to experience across the lifespan adds a note of hopefulness to the treatment of early relational trauma in later childhood and adolescence, although the earlier the timing of the original experience, the less malleable to change (Perry et al., 1995).

Furthermore, understanding the inter-play between child development and environment can better inform our understanding of process in therapeutic interventions with children who might be struggling to overcome developmental and social difficulties. The insights gained from understanding the place for humanity in the reciprocal community between species in the natural environment, and the mothering role of the oldest trees in the woodland, provides possibilities in therapy for extending the developmental, sensual, and emotional territory of childhood beyond the human family to include the environment as a therapeutic ally.

Nature-based therapeutic nurture group

To link theory to practice, the following vignettes drawn from my clinical experience are from an urban nature-based therapeutic nurture group, which describe how effectively young children can overcome their difficulties and find their own way into playing with their peers, when they feel safe in a playful and responsive environment, and are able to call on sensitive and timely therapeutic support from a developmental and trauma-informed play therapist. In the following illustrative examples, pseudonyms are used and any identifying information has been altered as well as including some composite case study material.

We had access to a local authority maintained woodland in the same locality of the school, but not within easy walking distance and separated by busy roads. The children (aged 4–5 years) were bussed there in two shifts for 3-hour sessions, morning and afternoon (total of 30 children). The 3-hour sessions provided the children with a predictable structure within which they could plan their own play agendas, with time for snacks and whole group coming together before the session ended. We provided a selection of tools and play materials to augment the natural materials to be found in the woodland. We carefully assessed the risk in the play areas before each session, removed any dangerous hazards, and made notes of lesser hazards that the children needed to be aware of. As part of our responsibilities towards the site, we were careful not to allow the woodland to become depleted; we would set up in a rotation of different areas to allow those areas impacted by our presence to settle and regenerate. We had a team of practitioners and volunteers, resulting in an overall ratio of 4 children: 1 adult. The child-centred ethos encourages free-flowing child-directed play, trusting the children in their ability to direct their own play and to assess risks as they play. With this level of self-reliance evident amongst most of the children most of the time, we were available to respond to cues from individual children in need of support.

Saul aged 4.5 years

At first, Saul was often on the edge of other children's play, watching. His difficulties included shyness, and impaired mobility and hearing. He took time to work out how to manage the unfamiliar woodland environment, watching the other children finding their way, imagining himself there with them but not quite ready yet to find his own way into joining them. For the first two sessions, he occasionally seeks eye contact with me for a moment, and then he turns away. Then one morning, he catches my eye and he hides behind a tree, and I find him. He is delighted to be found, and we repeat the game several times. Then he stops in a clearing and he starts to pile brash and sticks. Together we build what he names: "a wall to climb through", which he does, back and forth for the remainder of the session.

The next session he cues me in with eye contact, and he becomes affectionate and physically playful, mud painting me from behind. I am crouching, and he sits on my knees and begins a pushing game, enjoying the proprioceptive feedback of weight and pressure, the rhythm of resistance and yield. I attune to his touch, and he uses me to stand up. Some other children a few feet away have seen what we were doing and started their own version of the game. After a short while, he joins them.

Saul knew what he wanted to do, and where he wanted to be and he needed to find his own way, at his own pace, reaching out for support through the medium of play. In the initial stages, he stayed on the edge, imagining himself "over there, with them", and seeking ways to connect from his temporary isolation without losing himself. He needed to trust the ground beneath him before taking that step. Hide and seek is developmentally significant, the child communicating his need to be found, to be seen, and to be held in mind when he disappears. I was able to provide him a reminder of that felt sense of a significant (m)other in the moment of his uncertainty. So often we see children making sense and finding their way through play that meets their developmental needs at the moment, and often this means travelling back in time to an earlier stage that provides them with reassurance and co-regulation from another for the task ahead. Reading his play from a developmental perspective, we can see that Saul needed to build a trusting relationship with a significant adult in order to feel secure in this unfamiliar environment.

The woodland provides a rich source of loose parts, those material and ephemeral elements that inspire creative expression (Nicholson, 1971). I was struck by the symbolism of the stick wall for this child as he found his own way forward, and I was able to track his process and reflect back to him on the significance of his ability to build and climb through his "wall". He discovered that I was an adult who understood him, and he trusted my presence, finding that with me he could express his true self playfully in relationship with his environment: hiding behind trees, making use of sticks, messing with mud, and enjoying proprioceptive feedback and support. This was embodied play with a supportive adult in a rich and playful environment that oriented him and bridged the chasm between himself and his peers. He came from a secure and loving family and he already had the necessary "implicit relational knowing" (Stern, 1985) to reach out for connection. He was temporarily uncertain and overwhelmed by his environment and he found the support he needed to gain confidence and find his own way forward. Stern (2010) points out that changes occur only when one "does", i.e. moves and enacts. Mental models and neural networks can be re-patterned by doing something differently, imagining it differently, seeing another do it, or hearing about it: the vital thing is that all have to pass through imagination and movement, and play is the perfect medium for this alchemy.

Anny aged 4 years

We were told that Anny seldom spoke at school although she did speak at home. Initially, she never spoke to us. Occasionally she would grunt, squawk, or gesture if she needed something. Her play was noticeably solitary, although she kept within sight and hearing of the other children and she seemed interested in their play. Elective mutism and social anxiety are often correlated (Milic et al., 2020), and the combined effect can frustrate and suppress a child's urge to communicate and significantly impact their development and learning. Anny's anxiety prevented her from being herself in social situations. She could only reach out to others using animal noises: self-protection by imagining herself as something other than herself.

The animal puppets came in the play kit every session and were popular with the children and used in many different ways in their play. They were a catalyst for a significant breakthrough for Anny. Anny chooses Bee and Mosquito puppets, and she runs past and "stings" me, and then retreats behind a tree. I am holding Squirrel, and Squirrel peeps around the tree, making friendly noises. Anny is delighted. Later the same day, Anny has Squirrel peeping round trees at the other children, making little noises, and they respond to her. Over the next two months, she becomes gradually more integrated into group play, at first as a polar bear the other children "feed" and then as herself. Over a period of several months, we become increasingly aware that she is chatting with her friends.

Anny wants to join in with the other children but she struggles to connect with them. The woodland animal puppets provide a medium for her to project herself outwards, first into "stinging" characters, and she uses these to let me know through sound and gesture: "Here I am, I am not safe, I will sting you, come and get me". I respond, letting her know through Squirrel puppet: "Here I am, I am safe, I am friendly, I want to play with you". Through the medium of symbolic play, using movement and sound, Anny (as Bee and Mosquito) is able to tell me how she is feeling and what she wants, and I (as Squirrel) am able to respond with loving care, providing her with the transformative experience of being heard and understood. She experiences Squirrel being friendly and this provides her with the possibility of *being* friendly Squirrel. She tries this out, initiating interactions that bring her into playful connection with her peer group, first as Squirrel, then in the imaginative guise as their Polar Bear protégée, and then as her authentic self.

In many years of practice as a play-worker and child therapist, I have noticed that most children move easily back and forth across species boundaries, forming relationships with all forms of more-than-human life, including reptiles, invertebrates, plants, trees, mammals, marine life, and birds. The history of art and literature from all over the world is testament to human imagination as naturally anthropomorphic, and children exemplify this in their play (Griffiths, 2013). Many of their play narratives blur the boundaries between human and other-than-human, providing evidence of the flow of communication and identification between children and other species. This supports a felt sense of connection and, exploration of sameness and difference engenders a sense of belonging and a gateway to enter the spiritual life. There are social benefits in their play narratives, helping children to communicate their experiences, explore moral questions, and learn important life lessons.

Coda

Saul comes towards me with a stick in his hand, raised above his shoulder. "Javelinnnn!" he shouts as he sent the stick flying between the trees to my left. John is watching. He picks up another stick, runs, and throws it wildly in the same direction. Saul says "Come here, I'll show you how to do javelin". He throws again, and they take it in turns, keeping to their idiosyncratic throwing styles, throwing in the same direction. At first, I am the Commentator, giving my full attention, and a running commentary. Holly comes over, she takes a turn, then sits beside me and watches for a while, then counting them into the run and creating a pile of sticks, and a new rule: "You have to change that one for another one now". The boys throw, pick up, and exchange their sticks. Two more children, including Anny join in the play in an atmosphere of quiet concentration. My job now is to warn other children to watch out for flying sticks.

These vignettes demonstrate how nature becomes a therapeutic ally for the therapist and child, as each child overcomes their challenges to connect socially with their peers. The affordances of the woodland offered opportunities for responsive communication between the children, their environment, and a significant adult, providing developmentally appropriate support that encourages social connection through embodiment and imaginative play.

The play therapist's role in a nurture group is to prepare well, including being well informed about each child's developmental history, in order to be totally present for a complex task. During sessions, it is vital to pay careful attention to verbal, non-verbal, physical, and emotional use of self, as well as maintaining alert presence, engendering and maintaining the felt sense of containment for the group's autonomous and dynamic evolution, and to be available as a witness for individuals as they find their own way, tuning in to their own pace and way of being. It is so important too that our own relationships with the other-than-human world are intrinsic to our practice, so that we can follow the child's play, wherever they may lead us.

Nature-based Play Therapy

Many children, who are referred to our play therapy service, struggle to manage in group situations. The majority will have experienced disrupted early attachment and many sudden changes in chaotic and hostile environments. They may have been exposed to physical and emotional violence and neglect. Their experiences have taught them that their lived world is a frightening and untrustworthy place, and their sense of self may be isolated, fragmented, and incoherent (Winnicott, 1949; Schore, 2001). They may have developed coping strategies of avoidance, dissociation, or aggression (Perry et al., 1995). They may be impacted by the pervasive and devastating felt sense of core shame (Cozolino, 2014; Fearn, 2020). Many of these children will have a profound mistrust of adults, and their defensive patterns can be triggered by the intensity of one-to-one relationship in a closed play therapy room. Calling on nature as our therapeutic ally can provide the child with encounters that do not trigger the child's defences.

The following vignettes from one-to-one play therapy sessions demonstrate how nature can contribute to a child's process in Play Therapy. The sessions take place in a space that has been carefully designed to consider indoor/outdoor connectedness between the playroom and the enclosed outdoor woodland garden in relation to developing a close match between the stream of sensory information and opportunities for playful interaction through movement and touch experiences (Fearn, 2021). This sanctuary communicates to the child "You are safe; you can play here in any way you want to". At the same time, the presence of the play therapist communicates the following message: "You can play here in any way you wish. I am here to keep you safe and if there is anything you can't do, I will let you know". The messages from the play therapist and the Nature-based Play Therapy space coalesce into a continuous felt sense of security and containment that supports the child's expression of subjective reality in the shared play space, witnessed and validated by the play therapist. This provides an optimum environment for the child's therapeutic process and recovery. In the following illustrative example, a pseudonym is used and any identifying information has been altered as well as including some composite case study material.

Grace aged 7 years

Like many children who find themselves in local authority care, Grace's early years were chaotic and frightening. She came to play therapy presenting with hypervigilance, aggression, self-harming, and controlling behaviours that made her difficult to care for and which severely interfered with her attempts to make friends and connect socially with her peers. For our purposes, it is not necessary to tell the details of her life, that may have been known beforehand or revealed in her play, just sufficient to say that there was a parallel therapeutic process that enabled her to begin to develop a coherent narrative and to make sense of and express her feelings about what had happened to her. Rather, my intention is to focus on the evolution of her embodied therapeutic process and the role of nature as a therapeutic ally in extending the territory of the shared subjective play space between the play therapist and child.

Grace lets me know in our very first session that she hates spiders. She sorts through the sand tray miniatures to eliminate every spider and multi-legged insect she could find by throwing them across the room. This is done at great speed, as is everything else she does in these early sessions. Clearing up after that first session I search for the plastic anthropods and invertebrates Grace has thrown, and I return them to their place on the miniatures shelf. In the following sessions, she ignores them and never tries to evict them again. Over time her play themes multiply and diverge away from this initial focus for her deep-rooted and pervasive fear. The primary motivational drive to control her environment remains. In the early sessions, she rushes into and out of her play, using the inside and outside spaces with many disruptions and, for me, bewildering changes of direction. She rarely settles, and she explores every physical and emotional limit and boundary she can find, testing the trustworthiness of the play space and the play therapist, leaving me feeling anxious and with a panicky sense of trying to keep up. So often in Play Therapy does the child give us a felt sense of their experience of being in the world!

Although supported by many years' experience and a profound belief in the inherent Therapeutic Powers of Play, with Grace I need to remind myself often to trust the process, and I would reflect minutely on our sessions afterwards trying to find any evidence of a shift in theme or change in patterns of responding. Moments of change in play therapy can present in subtle and nuanced ways, such as barely noticeable shifts in energy, a change in proximity to the therapist, or a change in need for limit setting (Landreth, 2012). As she began to settle, her aggression lessens, and my role as "the stupid one who cannot keep up" shifts to becoming her accomplice, with "the stupid one" relegated to the status of a third imaginary presence. During this role-play, the limit setting I need to impose to keep us safely grounded in reality (physical and emotional) provides a brake on Grace's omnipotence and reminds her of our shared humanity. Gradually a kinder, more careful, and more balanced way of being in the world emerges between us.

The natural elements in the enclosed outdoor space become a significant therapeutic ally in Grace's therapeutic process, putting her in touch with sensory experiences her body is hungry for. She loves the swing on the little oak climbing tree, ordering: "Spin me!" this way, then that. I keep her within safe limits, watching her carefully for signs of overwhelm. She thrives on the vestibular stimulation and enjoys feeling dizzy, laughing as she stumbles about, trying to walk after spinning. When it rains, she runs onto the veranda to watch and listen to its rhythm drumming on the plastic roof. She dodges out into the rain, face to the sky, eyes closed, arms held out, and then dodges back under cover breathless with excitement, smiling straight at me, guileless. She leads this way and that way on adventures exploring the woodland and the stream beyond the garden, checking behind to make sure I am right there with her. As she plays with the natural space, I am consistently available, keeping her safe, and attuned to her, and I notice how in my presence, she is learning to trust herself.

Turning points in Play Therapy can also be sudden with a marked shift in energetic expression (Yasenik and Gardner, 2019). It is early Spring. Grace begins the session by playing in the Play Therapy room. Outside, the box trees and daffodils are in flower. The bumblebees, famished after their long winter sleep, are seeking out nectar. The air is warming. Grace takes the play outdoors, initiating a game of tag. We charge around the garden for a few minutes, using the central flowerbed as a roundabout in our chase game. Grace stops to take a breath, holding up her hand to pause the game, gasping "Freeze!". I keep still. The daffodils distract her, and she gazes deep into a yellow trumpet. She jumps suddenly when a bumblebee flies past her ear and lands on the daffodil trumpet she was gazing into. Fascinated she watches the creature walk in and emerge covered in yellow pollen to fly off, and without hesitation, Grace's nose enters the daffodil's trumpet to emerge a moment later dipped in yellow pollen. She stands quietly with her eyes closed, breathing deeply. The session is coming to an end, and I give her the five-minute signal. She stays calm, leaving without her usual resistance to endings and with a dab of yellow pollen on the tip of her nose.

During the sessions that follow, Grace climbs the small oak climbing tree, embracing the moss-covered trunk with her whole body, testing her weight on each branch, stretching to the limits of her physical reach. The tree channels her impulsive chaotic energy into thoughtful balanced sensual movements. She climbs up and lounges on a branch for a while. Climbing down is always more challenging, and she needs to take her time, testing her foothold, keeping herself safe, as I stand beneath paying careful attention and tracking her every move. When the sun comes out, she tries to catch the comma butterflies on the asters, dazzled by the colour and movement. She is quick and focused, and she catches one by its wing between finger and thumb. I set the limit, reminding her of our agreement to do no harm, and immediately she releases it and it flutters away.

As she develops embodied awareness of her responses to the flow of sensory information from her environment and begins to integrate regulatory capacity, she is able to remain calm and present for longer periods of time and there is less aggression or dissociation. Her need to control everything diminishes. By late summer, there is a marked change noticed at home and in school. She is concentrating for longer periods; she is able to stop and think before action; she is beginning to show consideration for others; she is also enjoying group activities that satisfy her competitive spirit and love of movement. She is developmentally on track.

In therapy, Grace involves me more often in role-play as she explores her past experiences and tries to make sense of her world. One afternoon she is on the floor of the play therapy room and she stops and stares. There is one of the small plastic fly figures I had missed from her first session, caught in a crack in the floorboard. I pay careful attention and I quietly track her movements. After a moment, she moves on and her play takes another direction, but she seems more thoughtful and deliberate in her decision-making. In the following session, she arrives with a plan. Without preamble, she fetches a chair, drags it across the room against the wall, and tells me to hold her legs. She climbs onto the chair and with me holding her, she stretches up and touches a spider's web. In late summer, the delicate, long-legged house spider *pholcidae* occupies corners of the playroom. They create tangled inverted webs and wait for hours upside down for prey to land. The supersensitive hairs on their legs pick up the slightest movement, and they gyrate at great speed, spinning their prey into a web trap. When Grace touches the web the spider spins frantically, Grace screams and I feel her legs vibrate with the shock. She does not give up. Again and again, she reaches up to the web, saying "come on spider, come here". The spider retreats from her at great speed, changing direction and gyrating madly. Eventually, she sighs and climbs down, moving the chair around the room to approach other spiders. As she does so she slows down, her breathing deepens and she moves more carefully. At last, she is rewarded when a spider moves across her hand. It makes her jump and she shrieks and laughs, she follows the spider, exhorting it to "come back!" She fetches the plastic fly and attempts to "feed" it to the spider.

Porges (2007) tells us that our nervous system constantly scans our surroundings. Hanna agrees: "Every millimetre of our body surface is in the business of perceiving and thus every portion of our bodily surface is conscious. Our whole sensitive body is conscious; it is constantly attentive to stimuli" (1970: 79). Until this session, Grace had given no indication that she had noticed the spiders on their webs in the playroom. Weeks later, in her final session, she is delighted to find a spider in her play therapy box. She announces proudly this proves that the spider wants to come home with her.

Reflecting on Grace's process encourages us to focus on sensory integration in Nature-based Play Therapy. There is evidence of her gradually increasing awareness of being balanced and physically in control and the remarkable development of her self-regulatory capacity that leads to emotional healing. It is argued elsewhere that access to sensory play and nature is a necessary prerequisite for sensory integration (Fearn, 2014; Prendiville and Fearn, 2017). Grace's therapeutic journey shows us that nature can be a powerful therapeutic ally for supporting the healing of a traumatised child whose sense of self was fragmented and incoherent, and who was prey to the agony of sensory and emotional overwhelm in her autonomic nervous system that is the legacy of relational trauma and abuse (van der Kolk, 2014).

In his theory of human cognition, Piaget (1977) speculated on a constant human biological drive towards equilibrium, when the functions of assimilation and accommodation are in balance. Hanna notes that "this is the optimum state of human balance in its constant intercourse with the environing world" (1970: 114). This resonates with the concept of the biological drive to maintain homeostasis in regulation theory, arriving at the calm resting state of the regulated nervous system (Schore, 2005). Psychological and biological theories complement each other and provide a compelling theoretical support for the concept of "self actualisation" in psychotherapy as a somatic as well as psychological phenomenon (Maslow, 1943; Rogers, 1961), and furthermore, to conceptualise it as an optimum baseline state, rather than a pinnacle of achievement.

Drawing on the therapeutic powers of play and in triangulated dynamic relationship with her play therapist and nature, Grace experienced the flow between modalities of perception in a playful somatic relationship, grounding her in a sense of place and supporting her to discover an embodied sense of self. This is the firm ground in the present moment from which she can look back over her shoulder at that which came before and begin to imagine a future for herself.

Children who have been profoundly betrayed by those who should have loved and cared for them as infants need time and support that is trauma informed and developmentally sensitive. At her own pace and in her own way, Grace overcame the pervasive fear that had been driving her frantic attempts to live her life. As her tolerance expands, the fear diminishes, and through the medium of play, she manages her own gradual exposure to overcome her phobia and develop a playful relationship with spiders.

Conclusion

The multi-dimensional relationship between child, environment, and play therapist evolves through play, and the vignettes demonstrate that aspects of the therapeutic relationship can serve either as a timely reminder of secure attachment experiences, as shown in the case of Saul, or as a reparative alternative, giving the child experience of attuned attention, regulation and care, and opening up the possibilities for development of different relational patterns, as seen in Grace's case. Through attunement with an attentive adult and with access to the symbolic powers of play, Anny experienced being met, and being understood and accepted by her peers on her own terms and then as an equal social actor. Play is not only a process that promotes growth and development but is also the therapeutic medium for children to recover from trauma and heal (Parson, 2021). The therapeutic change agents inherent in the examples from clinical practice presented here demonstrate that play in nature facilitates authentic self-expression, fosters recovery from deep hurt, increases personal strengths, including embodied confidence and efficacy, and enhances social relationships, including peer friendships (Schaefer and Drewes, 2014).

The richness and diversity offered by the natural community in all three cases support interconnectivity and multiple channels of communication between the child, environment, and therapist. It is augmented by the play therapist's ability to utilise their presence and competence to offer a consistent felt sense of safety and containment that supports the child's process. The role of the play therapist is to witness and reflect the child's process as they manifest their authentic and essential selves, to restore their right to a core belief in the coherence and consistency of existence between inner and outer worlds, which allows the child to trust in her self and her experiences in and of the world "out there" from the perspective of an embodied sense of self. The child's propensity to play with modalities of perception and undergo profound developmental change is evident if they feel safe, seen, and cared for in a multi-sensory and responsive environment. Children want to be healthy and they want to play, and both are a human right and enshrined in Welsh Government legislation (Convention on the Rights of the Child, 1989). *The Big Ask: The Big Answer* report 2021 reveals that children want to escape the digital labyrinth in which they feel trapped. The report tells us that they want to be outside – to be in open spaces, and play (de Souza, 2021). Emotional health, optimum development, healing from trauma and true sustainability reside in acknowledging that environmental connection is a survival issue and is an embodied, somatic experience: reconnecting body and earth through the medium of play is not only possible, but it is also vital.

References

11 Million (2008) *Fun and freedom: What children say about play in a sample of play strategy publications*, London: Children's Commissioner for England.

Anda, R.F., Felitti, R.F., Walker, J., Whitfield, C., Bremner, D.J., Perry, B.D., Dube, S.R. and Giles, W.G. (2006) 'The enduring effects of childhood abuse and related experiences: A convergence of evidence from neurobiology and epidemiology', *European Archives of Psychiatric and Clinical Neuroscience*, 256(3), 174–186.

Aposhyan, S. (2004) *Body-mind psychotherapy: Principles, techniques and practical applications*, New York, NY: W.W. Norton & Co.

Convention on the Rights of the Child (1989) available: https://gov.wales/childrens-rights-in-wales [accessed 12 December 2021].

Cozolino, L. (2014) *The neuroscience of human relationships. Attachment and the developing social brain*, 2nd edn., New York, NY: Norton & Norton.

Csikszentmihalyi, M. (1990) 'Flow: The psychology of optimal experience', *Journal of Leisure Research*, 24(1), 93–94.

de Souza, R. (2021) *The big ask: The big answers*, report by Children's Commissioner for England, September 2021, available: www.childrenscommissioner.gov.uk/the-big-answer/ [accessed 9 January 2021].

Fearn, M. (2014) 'A natural space for healing: Working therapeutically with groups outdoors', in E., Prendiville and J., Howard (eds.) *Play therapy today: Contemporary practice for individuals and groups*, Oxon: Routledge.

Fearn, M. (2020) 'The seeds of shame: The developmental impact of persistent misattunement in infancy', *British Journal of Play Therapy*, 13, 6–19.

Fearn, M. (2021) 'Integrating the therapeutic powers of play in nature-based play therapy', in E., Prendiville and J., Parson (eds.) *Clinical applications of the therapeutic powers of play: Case studies in child and adolescent psychotherapy*, Oxon: Routledge.

Fearn, M. and Troccoli, P. (2017) 'Being, becoming and healing through movement and touch', in E., Prendiville and J., Howard (eds.) *Creative psychotherapy. Applying the principles of neurobiology to play and expressive arts based practices*, Oxon: Routledge.

Griffiths, J. (2013) *Kith: The riddle of the childscape*, London: Hamish Hamilton.

Hanna, T. (1970) *Bodies in revolt. A primer in somatic thinking*, New York, NY: Holt, Rheinhart and Winston.

Jennings, S. (1999) *Introduction to developmental playtherapy: Playing and health*, London: Jessica Kingsley Publishers.

Laevers, F. (1993) 'Deep level learning: An exemplary application on the area of physical knowledge', *European Early Childhood Education Research Journal*, 1, 53–69.

Landreth, G.L. (2012) *Play therapy: The art of the relationship*, 3rd edn., New York, NY: Routledge.

Maslow, A.H. (1943) 'A theory of human motivation', *Psychological Review*, 50(4), 370–396.

Merleau-Ponty, M. (2012/1945) Phenomenology of perception, Donald Landes (trans.), London: Routledge.

Milic, M.I., Carl, T. and Rapee, R.M. (2020) 'Similarities and differences between young children with selective mutism and social anxiety disorder', *Behaviour Research and Therapy*, 133, 1–11.

Nicholson, S. (1971) 'How not to cheat children: The theory of loose parts', *Landscape Architecture Quarterly*, 62, 30–34, re-printed in *Ip-Dip. For Professionals in Play*, 9, May 2009.

Norwood, F.N., Lakhani, A., Fullagar, S., Maujean, A., Downes, M., Byrne, J., Stewart, A., Barber, B. and Kendall, E. (2019) 'A narrative and systemic review of the behavioural, cognitive and emotional effects of passive nature exposure on young people: Evidence for prescribing change', *Landscape and Urban Planning*, 189, 71–79.

Parson, J.A. (2021) 'Children speak play. Landscaping the therapeutic powers of play', in E., Prendiville and J., Parson (eds.) *Clinical applications of the therapeutic powers of play. Case studies in child and adolescent psychotherapy*, Oxon: Routledge.

Perry, B.D. (2001) 'The neuroarcheology of childhood maltreatment: The neurodevelopmental costs of adverse childhood events', in B., Geffner (ed.) *The cost of child maltreatment: Who pays? We all do*, San Diego: Family Violence and Sexual Assault Institute.

Perry, B.D., Pollard, R.A., Blakley, T.L., Baker, W.L., Vigilante, D. (1995) 'Childhood trauma, the neurobiology of adaptation, and "use-dependent" development of the brain: How "states" become "traits"', *Infant Mental Health Journal*, 16(4), 271–291.

Piaget, J. (1977) 'Problems of equilibration', in M.H., Appel and L.S., Goldberg (eds.) *Topics in cognitive development*, Boston, MA: Springer.

Porges, S.W. (1995) 'Orienting in a defensive world: Mammalian modifications of our evolutionary heritage: A polyvagal theory', *Psychophysiology*, 32, 301–318.

Porges, S.W. (2007) 'The polyvagal perspective', *Biological Psychology*, 74(2), 116–143, Doi: 10.1016/j.biopsycho.2006.06.009.

Prendiville, E. (2021) 'The EPR informed psychotherapist', in E., Prendiville and J., Parson (eds.) *Clinical applications of the therapeutic powers of play. Case studies in child and adolescent psychotherapy*, Oxon: Routledge.

Prendiville, S. and Fearn, M. (2017) 'Coming alive: Finding joy through sensory play', in E., Prendiville and J., Howard (eds.) *Creative psychotherapy. Applying the principles of neurobiology to play and expressive arts based practices*, Oxon: Routledge.

Rodaway, P. (1994) 'Sensuous geographies: Body, sense and place, London: Routledge, cited in Bartos, A.E. (2013) 'Children sensing place', *Emotion, Space and Society*, 9, 89–98.

Rogers, C.R. (1961) *On becoming a person*, Boston: Houghton Mifflin.

Schaefer, C.E. and Drewes, A.A. (eds.) (2014) *The therapeutic powers of play: 20 core agents of change*, Hoboken, NJ: John Wiley & Sons.

Schore, A.N. (2001) 'The effects of early relational trauma on right brain development, affect regulation, and infant mental health', *Infant Mental Health Journal*, 22, 201–269.

Schore, A.N. (2005) 'Back to basics: Attachment, affect regulation, and the developing right brain: Linking developmental neuroscience to paediatrics', *Paediatrics in Review*, 2(6), 204–217.

Simard, S. (2013) *Finding the mother tree. Discovering the wisdom of the forest*, London: Allen Lane.

Stern, D.N. (1985) *The interpersonal world of the infant. A view from psychoanalysis and developmental psychology*, New York, NY: Basic Books.

Stern, D.N. (2010) *Forms of vitality. Exploring dynamic experience in psychology, the arts, psychotherapy, and development*, Oxford: Oxford University Press.

Straus, E. (1966) *Phenomenological psychology*, London: Tavistock Publications.

van der Kolk, B. (2014) *The body keeps the score. Brain, mind and body in the healing of trauma*, New York, NY: Penguin Books.

Wilson, E.O. (1984) *Biophilia*, Boston: Harvard University Press.

Winnicott, D.W. (1949) *Mind and its relation to the psyche-soma*, London: Routledge.

Winnicott, D.W. (1991) *Playing and reality*, New York, NY: Psychology Press.

Yasenik, L. and Gardner, K. (2019) 'Turning points and understanding the development of self through play therapy', in L., Yasenik and K., Gardner (eds.) *Turning points in play therapy and the emergence of self. Applications of the play therapy dimensions model*, London: Jessica Kingsley Publishers.

7 Play and expressive arts to enhance professional development and personal growth in challenging contexts

Claudio Mochi, Steve Harvey, and Isabella Cassina

Section 1 introduces the contiguum *of professional development-personal growth by pre-senting the basic components of a multi-phased approach in the framework applied to a project in India. This approach is supported by a diagram showing how the two processes of professional development and personal growth reinforce each other with the first giving progressively more space to the second. Section 2 focuses on creative collaborations between therapists in co-creating metaphors and overcoming shared challenges and discomfort. Two examples are provided: the first presents an online play space dedicated to professionals from around the world. The second is related to a supervision group in New Zealand who faced a difficult situation at work and decided to find new answers and meanings through an arts-based inquiry.*

In the previous chapters, the reader would appreciate the application of the therapeutic powers of play, play therapy methodologies, and expressive arts in a multitude of complex and dynamic contexts and different cultures, both in-person and online, inside and outside the playroom. Contemporary world circumstances are more complex than the referrals from more traditional contexts and times (see Chapter 1 on the assumption of an increasing complexity and duration of crises). The emotional atmosphere can be confused, hostile, and filled with suffering. The emerging process and techniques used by professionals need to be current and co-created by all actors involved to have relevance.

Professionals working with children, adolescents, and families are required to be flexible and creative in expanding their awareness and understanding of the context and evolving new priorities, adapting and widening their skills, and using and integrating a variety of approaches to meet clients' needs and structural conditions. In this chapter, the authors focus on the role of play and expressive arts to enhance (among other abilities) creativity for professionals in the moments before and after the direct work with clients. Examples of projects from around the world will be provided starting from three assumptions:

1 "In sitting with and treating the suffering of others every day, we [professionals/ therapists] are exposed to pain and trauma and the inevitable effects it has on our nervous systems and bodies" (Bush cited in Gil, 2020). The effort to adjust to emerging difficult situations, the amount of work that extends

DOI: 10.4324/9781003252375-8

outside the therapeutic space, and the dealing with unpredictable and upsetting circumstances may challenge professionals' adaptive responses and affect their effectiveness and wellbeing. Some may be severely distressed and come to perceive "feelings of depression, hopelessness, and inadequacy" (McCann and Pearlman cited in Ryan and Cunningham, 2007: 447). Professionals "are containers for story after story of unhappiness and human struggle, with a never-ending responsibility to hold the tragic secrets of others" (Bush op. cit.). Regular exposure to the context of suffering may produce an "alteration in professionals cognitive schemas" affecting their sense of security and vulnerability (McCann and Pearlman, op. cit.). Professionals may reach the point where they doubt their own role as agents of change, all the more so if they themselves are experiencing critical circumstances;

2   Play and expressive arts have transformative and healing powers that can be expanded and fit contemporary new challenges. Individuals can learn how to use them as a transformative process and feel "as a creative participant in life" (Halprin, 1999: 137). "The fulfillment of experiencing one's own creativity through [play and] art-making lends courage and motivation to the task of confronting and releasing destructive life experiences" (op. cit.). The potential of transformation and healing can be applied to both individual and group (or community) challenges. Rogers (1999: 116–117) underlines how "two major healing elements of the expressive arts process [are]: first, the changes that happen in the creative act itself; and second, the growth and insight that occurs when we study the image or the process for its meaning".

3   Play and expressive arts are fundamental resources in the *contiguum* professional development-personal growth. Landreth (cited in Blanco et al., 2014: 45) stated in this regard that "the most significant resource the therapist brings to the play [expressive] therapy relationship is the dimension of self. Skills and techniques are useful tools, but therapist's use of their own personalities is their greatest asset". From a timeline perspective, play and expressive arts enhance professionals' resources and abilities. This can support the professional for what comes before, during, and after the therapy sessions with clients. Play and expressive arts support professionals' acquisition of skills and techniques and nourish the development of both professional and personal self.

We will soon describe the experience of a project in India pointing out the characteristics of a multi-phased process for resources development based on play and expressive arts. Play and expressive arts are also critical in the supervision phase, as we can observe in the examples provided in Section 2. Within the context of supervision or peer-group work, play and expressive arts (and the subsequent development of creativity) can facilitate the process of sharing, understanding, making meaning, and developing solutions. This process is applicable to different scenarios such as the discussion of clinical cases, working on group dynamics, or dealing with situations outside work that affect the participants in the group.

Section 1: capacity building as a *contiguum* professional development-personal growth

> When faced with the large wall of a stressor, it is great if there emerges one singular solution that makes the wall crumble. But often, a solution instead will be a series of footholds of control, each one small but still capable of giving support, that will allow you to scale the wall.
>
> (Sapolsky, 2004)

Successful therapies are seldom the result of one brilliant solution and more often the combination of multiple factors and events that require clinical skills, effective methodologies, and techniques, together with refined professional abilities and specific personal qualities. McNiff (cited in Levine, 2005: 172) noted that in academic settings there is a tendency to ignore or minimise the student's personal growth as part of the educational experience, but he considers that aspect (the "personhood") as prominent in the training. In fact, it is people who change people (Perry and Szalavitz, 2017: 85) and the use of self and the reliance on personal qualities is necessary and inevitable in therapeutic work.

> On the way to becoming a play [expressive arts] therapist, one must understand oneself, one's own beliefs, attitudes, values, the qualities of one's being, the nature of one's life, one's internal proclivities, resources, and tendencies, and external talents and skills. To know oneself in truth and fully is the direct path to being receptive to and knowing others.
>
> (Moustakas cited in Blanco et al., 2014: 48)

To summarise, professional development and personal growth are deeply intertwined and mutually enriching, and both are needed in working with clients, particularly in challenging contexts. Section 1 describes how these two elements are nurtured within a learning program using play and expressive arts. Figure 7.1 illustrates their evolution in the framework of a capacity-building process.

The diagram and the proportion of its elements (i.e. the triangles) are symbolic and meant to illustrate the following considerations:

- The initial step of the capacity-building process, as intended by the authors of this section, is the warm-up (this moment is explained later in the section). The warm-up provides the conditions that "help people to learn and to be open to the experiences" (ASCD Yearbook Committee, 1962: 143).
- Both professional development and personal growth are present from the beginning although in different proportions (we call this interweaving "*contiguum*").

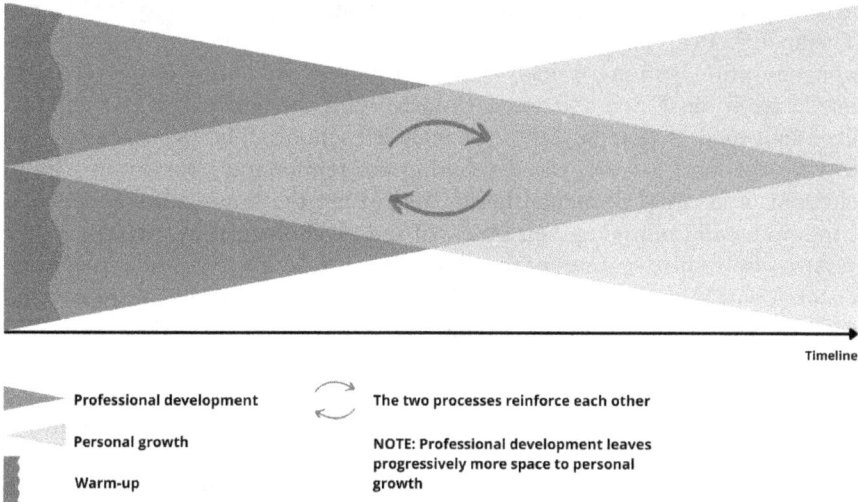

Figure 7.1 The evolution of the focus on professional development and personal growth in a capacity-building process.

Source: Diagram created by Isabella Cassina and Claudio Mochi.

- The learning of new cognitions, skills, and techniques is prevalent at the beginning and tends to decrease with time in favour of internal processes (such as affective modulation, self-awareness, self-exploration), and development of professional abilities (flexibility, creativity, playfulness, expressiveness, etc.). As time progresses, more and more attention and space are given to personal growth.
- Initially, the process is externally directed. Over time, it becomes progressively more self-directed by the practitioners/students. Skills, technical tools, and work guided by internal processes aim to build a base to expand possibilities for future exploration and discoveries (ASCD Yearbook Committee, 1962: 153–154).
- Along the *contiguum* professional development-personal growth, the space in the centre underlines the contingency and close connection between the professional and the person. It is difficult to indicate clearly where the professional ends and the person begins and vice versa (for the end result, does it really matter?). At this stage, the bottom line is that certain processes, abilities, and skills must be built, supported, and encouraged. Fostering self-understanding, developing awareness, and so on are all processes whose development benefits the client, the professional, and the person. The same applies to some personal abilities such as creativity, playfulness, and flexibility. These aspects need to be triggered, practised, and cultivated as they have an impact both inside and outside the playroom.

In 2018, we (Claudio and Isabella) were asked by a local organisation based in a rural area of India to conduct a project oriented to capacity building in Therapeutic Play. The project involved 58 local professionals from rehabilitation, education, and social fields working with 495 children with special needs, intellectually disability, and some children with cerebral palsy. The children lived in a total of nine facilities that included schools. The main goal, agreed to with the local partner, was developing and reinforcing a variety of skills in children in all areas of mental health, decreasing the limits imposed by their condition, and improving their potential and psychological wellbeing.

Apart from the diagnoses of the children, it is relevant to consider that more factors contributed to the vulnerability of all beneficiaries in the project. In particular, the risk class of the Country is "high" (INFORM Risk Index 5,2 out of 10; IASC and EC, 2021), the geographical area of the project is very poor (see considerations in Chapter 5), and some of the professionals suffered from physical disabilities due especially to poliomyelitis. It was clear from the beginning of our needs assessment that the project could not be limited to teaching new skills and techniques to implement with children. Something more complex and deep was needed, something that professionals could use in multiple circumstances in order to expand their own possibilities of wellbeing in a challenging and unpredictable context.

Our assessment was shown to be accurate and the process more than adequate and useful because since 2020, the pandemic (Covid-19) added countless factors of vulnerability. Unfortunately, the project has been temporarily suspended, as most of the children and professionals moved from the area to rejoin their families and the international borders closed. No one could have foreseen the timing nor the magnitude of this Covid 19 crisis, but the foundation set in our training allowed professionals to continue applying the skills and methodologies learned as soon as they were back to work. Let's explore how the capacity-building process was developed in that context.

Phase 1

Initially, the therapeutic powers of play and expressive/creative arts were used to assess the needs, to start building a relationship and a feeling of trust with the trainers and participants. As a starting point, an introductory training to the main field (such as Play Therapy) proved to be an ideal circumstance to address the needs of the three main actors: the professionals (or participants of the training program), the trainers, and the local partner.

During the introductory training (generally three to six full days), the *professionals/participants* are the centre of attention. They feel valued, they have fun and relax while interrupting their complex and bittersweet routine with the children. They begin developing new ideas, recognise the feeling of belonging to the group by sharing experiences and emotions, and, last but not least, if we create the right atmosphere, they can start expanding their own playfulness and creativity. On paper, our introductory training in India included the following main goals: describe the value of play for individuals of all ages, list the distinctive elements of the play therapy field, identify at least seven benefits of using play with children for educational and therapeutic purposes, and practice playful and creative activities. But the training days included much more than this thanks to the involvement of the professionals in multiple activities that we (as trainers) suggested, modified, and co-created with them in an ongoing process.

In fact, during the introductory training, the *trainers* can: assess local professionals' needs and familiarity with specific topics and skills, collect more information on children's needs through professionals, start building an atmosphere of trust and safety by using specific interaction skills and play/expressive activities, get to know the participants individually, and discover their point of view on multiple topics. At the same time, the trainers can collect more information on the local culture and this specific group and refine their vocabulary and the timing of training activities in order to become more attuned with the group. Most importantly, they can start modelling the contents of the whole training and supervision program.

The *local partner*'s needs are fundamental too and the introductory training addresses a large part of their request. The Institution in India was a large organisational outfit providing human resources, spaces, and time. They wanted to see that the project was starting "for real", that something was already happening and that this first phase was more than "just an observation" from the trainers' side. Nonetheless, observing both children and professionals in the facilities and school is part of the ongoing assessment throughout the process. Also, the participants felt involved, motivated, and thankful, and the positive general mood was very well perceived by the board. The partner's needs have to be considered and honoured because without a partner wanting the project and believing in it as we do, there is no project at all.

Before introducing phase 2, we would like to share an activity from our introductory trainings: "Peanut butter/jelly game" (Munns, 2000: 293). Our project in India involved mainly occupational therapists and teachers working with mild to severe developmentally handicapped children and children with cerebral palsy. The particularity of our local partner is to employ some of their personnel who have physical handicaps such as walking difficulties and limb malformation and in some cases, deafness. For this reason, the activities we offered during the training were carefully selected and included a range of options for participants, especially when activities included movement.

In order for participants to fully understand the potential of the activities they were learning and would consequently share with their clients, we always invite them to experience the activities first hand. This allows us to achieve multiple goals such as conveying new ideas (including how to lead the activity) and also start stimulating participants' inclination to play and be creative. In other words, explaining an activity or reading it from a book allows us to learn it, while experiencing it first hand allows us to benefit actively from the emotion of play and, with time, to acquire the ability to develop further skills such as creating new activities and adapt them to the target audience.

"What is it that you like to eat?", most of them answered "Chapati and rice!". This is how I (Isabella) introduced the activity and the group renamed it. I invited my colleagues to listen to the way I was saying "chapati" and look at the movement I did and respond with "rice" using the same tone of voice and doing the same movement. They could stay seated or stand and move according to their ability and motivation. I started by whispering "chapati"; I smiled and waited for their reaction. They were all sitting and looking at me with a questioning look. I repeated: "chapati" and put the hand to my ear as if to hear their answer better. At that point, I heard the first silent answers: "rice". I smiled, I was getting them. I tried something louder with a slightly bigger and funny movement using both arms. More people answered, I started seeing the first smiles on their faces and hearing some shy laughter. I suggested they could stand up if they wanted to. I was astonished when most of them stood up regardless of their physical difficulties. I now felt that I had their full involvement and I could be a little more daring. After a few more preparatory steps, my voice was much louder, my movements bigger, the sequences were gradually longer. I was now saying: "Cha-cha-chaaapaaatiii" and I turned around and moved my hands up and down multiple times! Suddenly, Claudio and my Indian colleagues started laughing so much, an atmosphere of fun exploded in the room. We were there, all together, actively involved, without judgments nor worries about how we appeared. We were playing. We were putting aside for a moment the thoughts of working in a highly stressful situation while starting to build new awareness and skills for the future.

In the beginning, the activities should be fun, simple, short, possibly include movement, and (always) culturally appropriate. The trainers must be able to modify the activity in response to the immediate reaction of the participants. It is advisable to always have two trainers as well as groups up to a maximum of 25 people at a time for introductory trainings. Much smaller groups are recommended for advanced trainings and group supervision.

Phase 2

After phase 1, more training and experiential activities are planned to support professionals in acquiring new knowledge on specific topics and to start working on selected skills and capacities such as self-awareness and stress management. One of the modules we organised had the following main learning objectives: identify at least five reasons why play is fundamental for children with disabilities, discuss how to recognise and promote "true play" (Stagnitti, 2021), select toys and materials, prepare the playroom, and practice playful and creative activities. In further training, professionals discussed (pre-)pretend play as a "melting pot of abilities" (op. cit.) for children, how to recognise and stimulate it, and develop specific abilities.

As anticipated, all modules were accompanied by activities that go beyond learning skills, allowing the participants to elaborate and express their feelings, and to begin to understand various circumstances and how to cope with them.

Over time, the world of play and expressive arts became accessible to them and creativity a resource for them as professionals working with children. It also became personal as participants experimented, connected with each other, had fun and lots of laughter, and new possibilities opened up.

Phase 3

The next period of the training program is dedicated to the application of knowledge and new skills in the sessions with children and adolescents. In other words, we move inside the playroom. This is done physically if it is an option or alternatively through a video camera if it is not appropriate or feasible for the trainers to be there too. At this level, the trainers support the professionals both by doing live simulations and by modelling the work with children and providing individualised feedback. In phase 3, group and individual supervision on the application of new skills and methodologies and case management are included.

The process may seem to be over, but in reality, this is the beginning of a new cycle. In fact, seven steps in a circular fashion are planned (Mochi and Cassina, 2018), where the needs' assessment is ongoing and individual and group supervision highlights further training. The seven steps are as follows:

1   *Needs assessment:* how is the local support system organised? What do children and families need from the psychological point of view? What are professionals' resources and limits in order to meet these needs?
2   *Training:* is a practical response to the needs assessment considering the trainers' resources and limits. The training goes from generic to specific topics and includes theoretical and experiential components.
3   *Demonstration and shared activities:* the learning process moves into working spaces (classrooms, rehabilitation spaces, hospital rooms, etc.) where trainers model for the professionals new skills and play activities with children. Activities can also be co-conducted by trainers and professionals.
4   *Observations:* trainers observe the application of new skills and play activities by professionals and keep monitoring children. Trainers have an external role, they no longer model/guide the activities, but they do provide feedback to the professionals.
5   *Supervision:* is done individually and in groups, preferably by trainers viewing video recordings. Consent to record the sessions and play activities for professionals' education is always sought from the child's caregivers. If consent is not given, the supervision proceeds without recordings.
6   *Monitoring:* trainers verify the impact of the ongoing program on children, families, and professionals. Professionals monitor the impact on children and families. All data collected are necessary to adjust the ongoing training program or add new elements.
7   *New training and activities:* according to the results of the monitoring process and/or because of possible emerging needs, new training and activities can

be planned. If necessary, after step 7, a new cycle starts from step number 3 "demonstration and shared activities".

From steps 1 to 7, you will understand that trainers are not simply teaching new skills, but supporting their application, and tailoring and co-creating with the participants' further opportunities. As detailed in Chapter 1, this has many advantages such as building effective local human resources and reaching a bigger number of children and families. This process also gives the possibility for participants to start a transformative and beneficial process as "persons" (*vs.* professionals).

We would like to end Section 1 with an example of an activity developed with our colleagues in Venezuela. In 2017, we (Claudio and Isabella) were invited to Caracas by Doctors Without Borders to teach local professionals from the fields of mental health, education, and social work. The training program focused on how to use the therapeutic powers of play and play therapy to improve resilience and reduce stress reactions in children and adolescents in highly critical contexts. As a country, "Venezuela has one of the highest number of violent deaths in the region and in the world" (Overseas Security Advisory Council, 2020).

The activity was named "Un día en Caracas" (which means "one day in Caracas"; however, the country name can be substituted with any other that suits the purpose of the group). Participants are invited to break up into groups of three to five people and think about a typical day in their city. The second step is to agree on a general outline to be followed (no details, it just has to be a common idea or group "rules" to allow improvisation in the room). The key moments of the day are then enacted. Participants are provided disguises, puppets, and music instruments. This is what happened in Caracas:

> With a playful and ironic tone, women and men told a story about people waking up in Caracas in the morning to the sound of the alarm clock and hastily eating breakfast, giving way to pregnant women and the elderly on the bus, and trips on street-cars packed with people after waiting for hours. They enacted the fear of not arriving at work on time and being fired, entering a store and not finding flour and rice. They told stories of people who can't buy back the cell phone that was stolen from them, people who don't wear new earrings for fear of being robbed on the street, and people who are terrified of being kidnapped along the way and never being able to see their children again. Then there were families who go to church and hear gunshots and huddle on the ground remaining silent and shaking, and then come out of church and give a coin to a homeless person while making the sign of the cross.

After being on stage and seeing all the performances, we invited the groups to share their impressions and feelings about the whole experience and to give each scene a title agreed by the group. Lastly, we invited each participant to add an individual "aesthetic response" (Knill et al., 2005). Some of them made drawings, while others wrote short poems.

This kind of activity provides a safe space and time to express and explore experiences and emotions while unlocking the potential for creativity. In play, there is no "right" or "wrong"; there is no judgment nor limits to the imagination (Schaefer and Drewes, 2014). Through the scenes enacted, the participants could turn from being passive to being active. Having the feeling of control over the environment is an essential element in the development of positive mental health (Landreth, 1995: 46). The subsequent discussion and opportunity to provide an "aesthetic response" allowed the possibility to start raising awareness by "unpacking experiences" and formulating them in language in order to be re-integrated into the autobiographical story of each participant (McGilchrist, 2012; Mochi, forthcoming 2022).

The goal of improving resilience in children and adolescents also involves improving "the capacities [of professionals themselves] to deal effectively with stress and pressure; to cope with everyday challenges; to rebound from disappointments, mistakes, trauma, and adversity" (Brooks and Goldstein, 2015: 6). In this regard, we find confirmation in what Levine (1999: 33) mentions in his chapter, namely "I cannot relieve another human being of the burden of existence. Moreover, unless I have taken on the task of existence myself, I will be unable to show the way to anyone else".

Section 2: creative collaborations to co-create metaphors and overcome shared challenges and discomfort

In the capacity-building process described so far, the individual and group supervision component was particularly oriented to the application and refinement of new skills and case management (in both India and Venezuela, methodologies and techniques applied were related to the play therapy field). Less focus was on professionals' internal processes and self-growth. However, as presented in Figure 7.1, these components have been stimulated from the beginning through play and expressive arts. In fact, "supervision, like training in general, creates a challenging [and privileged] place for personal exploration" (Levine, 2005: 241–242).

The two examples provided in Section 2 illustrate the phase along the *contiguum* in which the process is more "internally" directed (by the participants themselves), and this leads to more opportunities to self-guide learning and discoveries. Both examples could be a way of continuing the process described in Section One (with the same group of professionals) or represent a stand-alone process (with another group of professionals for which the training component is not necessary). The projects described in this section will explore the dimension of supervision group and peer-group work oriented to internal processes, personal growth, and self-care. Particularly relevant is the co-creation of improvised metaphors as an expression of a common challenge and discomfort and as a starting point for an experience of hope and a shared solution.

The first project example is drawn from an international project to develop creative collaborations among therapists in different parts of the world during the current health crisis (Covid-19). This project (named for convenience "peer-group work") has not taken the form of a traditional therapy, supervision, or even support group but rather keeps becoming an emergent form that focuses participants on the shared creativity. In this example, the therapists address the emotionally volatile political situations and hostile emotional climate that has emerged in their communities around the public health policy in an online "play-space", which allows them to decentre from the problems they are facing (Levine, 2005: 239). In fact, "playing can relax and refresh as well as provide an opportunity to return to the material [or issue] with a new openness" (op. cit.).

The second project example was undertaken within a Creative Arts/Play Therapy supervision group to find a way to address a professional division within an agency around play approaches with young children during a time of budget restrictions. In both the situations described in this section, common understandings among those involved became challenged and the emotional cost of this conflict had become high. Over time, the online "play-space" and the supervision group created "a lively forum for dialogue, mutual support and connection" (op. cit.: 240).

Example 1: develop creative collaborations among therapists online

From 2020, the authors of this chapter have participated in a series of Zoom meetings led by Dr Steve Harvey in which a group of creative arts and play therapists from several countries have used a range of art modalities to develop improvisation with each other related to their experiences with the current global health crisis. As time has passed and with the development of social unrest, the themes of these improvised episodes have evolved to reflect new challenges than those presented in Chapter 2. This example emerged approximately 18 months after the initial session.

For the last several months, the social conflict and protest of the public measures related to vaccines and using masks have intensified. These protests have become very aggressive and even violent in many parts of the world. This social unrest often brings a hostile climate that surrounds all health and mental health-related activities including play and other creative arts therapy. Such aggression has included threats of violence towards some professionals in medical, mental health, and education sectors. This polarised social action has affected several members of the group of professionals, as many have ongoing work in schools, mental health clinics, and other medical agencies. Some of us live alongside protesters in our communities who express anger and even make threats to harm medical personnel and educators due to the requirement to become vaccinated or wear masks in the facilities in which we work.

This aggressive form of protest has occurred while young students, including children of our colleagues, and our colleagues themselves, have become seriously ill due to the virus while our professional positions and values have led us to continue to provide services. Some of us have experienced the death of our colleagues. In addition, all the members are from countries that have also recently had new surges in cases and deaths from the pandemic. This has placed some of us directly within a new social reality of hostility with few ways to escape. The surges have led to increased numbers of people seeking counselling and other related services. As the crisis has continued, several members of our group report approaching the point of physical and emotional exhaustion. These developments have increased our level of distress.

However, the creativity generated during our collaborations has contributed to the emergence of resiliency as reflected in the metaphors from the improvised dance, music, and fairytales and in the verbal reflections. As this protest, conflict, and alienation have developed, the group members through play and expressive arts have spontaneously generated images that reflect their experiences of the social unrest and complexity with some surprising results that include the experiences of hope. These collaborations have contributed to an alternative personal experience and shared good feeling that has helped members stand with more ease outside the current emotional reality of hostility and conflict.

The following improvisations were developed in a meeting during this time. This session began with a series of improvised dance and music duets followed by art and poetry making in response (see Figures 7.2–7.4). The dancers were cast from regions all over the world. Screens were spotlighted so that each

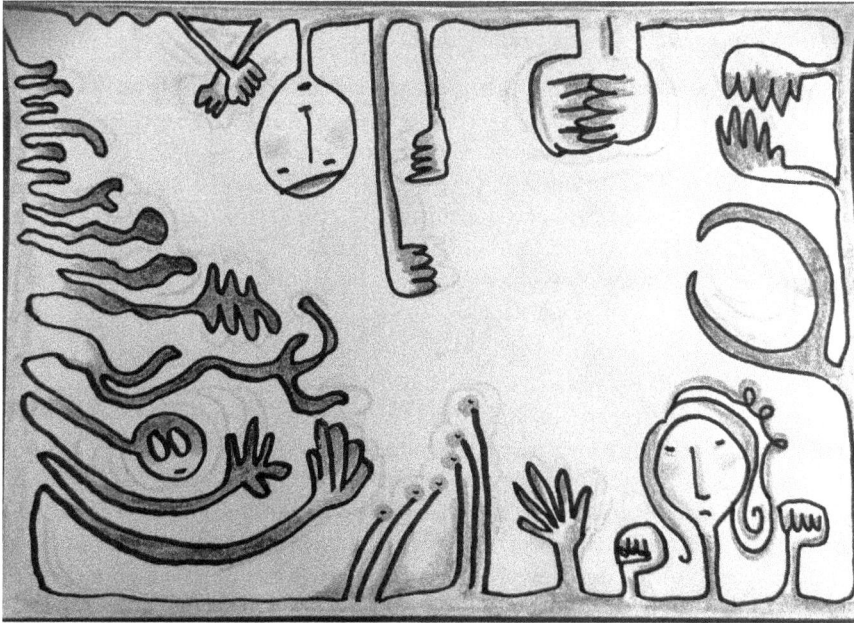

Figure 7.2 Art response to the duets.

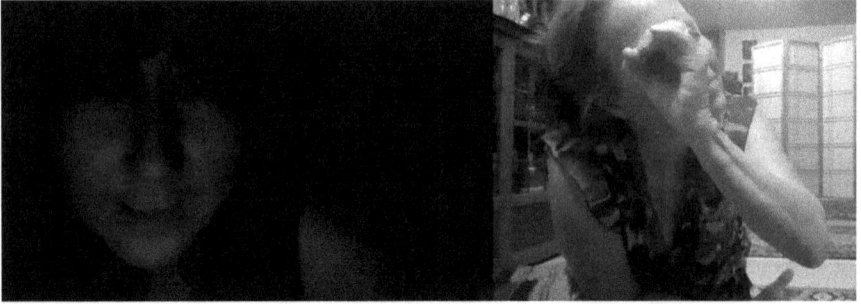

Figure 7.3 Picture of the final dance/fairytale.

person was next to each other as the only images in the larger view on the screen. This presentation suggested the metaphor of a global dance response to the current crisis. During these duets, members reported that the dances suggested imagery of the people fighting with Covid-19, people fighting in protest for their freedom, the conflict among different parts of our communities, the fight of our own internal fears, and a fight for our own emotional and physical life. As the metaphors developed, these expressions suggested a large range of simultaneous meanings.

A sample of poetic responses to these duets

The struggle exhausts us both. Yet goes on and on, there is no sunset on this.

Jagged edges, stalactites and stalagmites, the mountains and caves, to climb or descend. Caution and preparedness, readiness to step up or step down. Guarded passageways, unsure what path may unwind, to get us over, though, or next to, will burst or explode, or will we renew.

Fear and loneliness motivate our search. So painful to move nowhere. It is less if you search along the way.

This improvised expression helped transform the initial conversation about the anger, destructiveness, hostility, hopelessness, disruption of the protesters, and fear of becoming ill into larger symbols of the inner dilemmas of distress alongside hopes and fears for the future.

The final duet consisted of two dancers moving, while another member improvised a fairytale, and another responded with improvised vocal singing. In the scene, the dancers moved independently towards and away in relationship to each other from the edge of their screens. At one point, one of the dancers turned her light off and they both began to look for each other with one dancer in the dark. The scene ended with both dancers looking into their camera as if involved in an active search for each other.

The improvised fairytale told during the dance

The creatures began to move across the desert at midday. It grew warmer and warmer and warmer.

Towards the afternoon the winds came up and began to blow everything up – covering everything everywhere. The wind became a storm. The sand became blinding.

I don't like this. I don't want to be here.

How did I get here. I will stop this.

But they could not stop anything.

There must be some way forward. There must be someway backward. There must be someway underneath. There must be some way in the sky. There has to be.

In the darkness. In the nothingness.

I must reach out.

There you are. I never would have believed I could see something.

THERE, yes THERE!

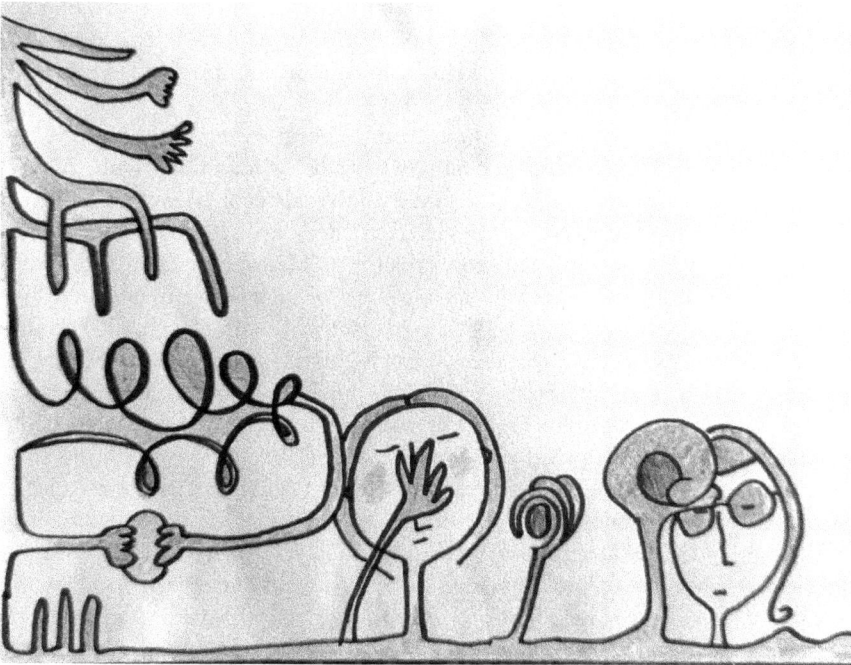

Figure 7.4 Art response to the fairytale.

Summary at the end of the session

> We are in the middle of global stress with our fellows, with Covid-19, with the future. We are in the middle of something with only occasional moments of light. Even a little less as we search to find something in the darkness. We find one another even in despair.

In the discussion following these improvisations, members acknowledged the difficult emotional experience of the current time and the important reference to hope within the improvisation mentioned at the end of the fairytale. The expressions of being overwhelmed, lost, and yet finding a positive feeling of being able to share these intimate experiences with each other through co-creativity was particularly important.

Example 2: develop a creative counter answer for complexity through supervision

This example is related to the dimension of a supervision group for mental health therapists in New Zealand. Harvey et al. (2016) reported about a supervision-related project that they developed to investigate change among young children and their families within a public mental health system. They undertook this project to help the therapists form a deeper understanding for the importance of their work as agents of change in which their agency challenged that relevance and had to marginalise them as important members of the larger service.

These therapists were part of a long-term ongoing supervision group. They were also part of a larger multi-disciplinary team (MDT) working with children and families who were referred to a Child and Adolescent Mental Health Service. This service was government designed, funded, and administered to address moderate to severe mental health concerns for problematic children and youth. Referrals came from community professionals. Presenting problems included children and youth with very low mood, anxiety, suicidal thinking and self-harming behaviours, threats of harm to others, and ongoing symptoms of psychological trauma associated with interpersonal or family violence and/or near-death experiences. Children and families among these referrals often presented with highly complex problems. Many had experienced several adverse events during their development. They were frequently unable to use verbal means to express and/or organise their distress and resisted attempts to introduce such methods. Such referrals were seen by the government as being among the highest need. The larger MDT was made up of professionals from psychiatry, psychology, social work, and mental health nursing. The team followed a traditional medical model. The child team addressed younger children and their families using play and expressive modalities when children were not able to use verbal therapies.

This team was set up to use standardised scales during intake in which behavioural problems related to categories such as emotional difficulty, harm to self and others, family, school, and social function were rated. The scales were used throughout the interventions and at the completion of treatments. These ratings were used to help determine diagnosis and treatment planning and to measure outcomes. Each referral case was presented to the MDT to determine the course, style, and length of treatment.

Prior to this project, the government had become concerned about waiting times and the number of referrals for service. A directive had been given to the team to favour shorter-term treatments. An unintended consequence of this was that creative and expressive approaches, which could be more tailored to specific children or families, were sidelined by the larger MDT. Results were to be reported in terms of changes in rating scores. The child's emotional changes reflected in creative metaphors that emerged from the expressive thera- pies became less valued. In turn, the play/expressive therapies and the creativity of the therapists who were engaged with the more non-verbal children became marginalised within the team. Play and other expressive action were actively discouraged despite the children's difficulty using verbal approaches. The for- mulations and progress reports presented to the MDT by the therapists were not considered as important by the overall service.

The supervision group decided that in addition to using the prescribed rat- ings, monitoring processes, and other MDT recommendations, they would try to understand how the play/expressive processes were able to impact the children and families they were asked to see. They essentially wanted to find out for them- selves what relevance the experiences of collaborative creative expression had for them as part of their supervision, rather than accepting the general negative tone about their approach from other professionals who had little to offer and no experience or interest in creative collaboration with these challenging cases.

The supervision group of therapists decided to develop a project using arts- based inquiry to investigate the changes they were observing. These changes were compared with the more traditional ratings required by the Ministry of Health. The group chose to intensively focus on a few cases involving chil- dren under ten and their families who had experienced significant family- related trauma, and who they had provided service for. Each of these children had shown some self-harming thought and behaviour. Two had witnessed and experienced family violence. One boy had attempted to use to knife to kill his mother and himself. The children were emotionally dysregulated and met the criteria for post-traumatic stress disorder and various types of mood and or anxiety disorders. Two of the children were prescribed medication with limited success. In each situation, the children were seen in both individual and fam- ily sessions, which used interactive expressive play. The expressive experiential modalities became the central component of treatment. To their credit, the larger team did agree that a medication only intervention would not be in these families' best interests. However, there was little interest or support for the use of play and creative expression.

Each child and family were able to engage in play activities such as sand tray, storytelling, improvised dance, and puppet dramas collaboratively with the therapists and family members. The children and their families showed improvement in every area of their functioning. Importantly, the children expressed an increase of shared positive feeling with their parents. Their self-harming and violent aggression towards themselves and their caretakers stopped. As the parents and children played together and listened to their stories, made puppet dramas, sand trays, and danced together, they were able to take charge of their lives again. This improvement occurred within a similar time frame to other patients of the service and with a similar number of sessions.

The supervision group wanted to find a way to investigate the subjective experience of what this change was like for the children, their families, and themselves in addition to and in parallel to the rating scale. They decided to employ an arts-based approach. Arts-Based Inquiry (McNiff, 1998; Hervey, 2000) is used to investigate complex questions which are difficult to address in other ways. The basic assumption of such inquiry is that important artistic expression can be produced when researchers have a close personal experience with issues being investigated within the project and that such an expression enhances the participants' overall awareness of their topic. By developing expressive metaphors, the non-verbal complexities of the changing shared emotional states could be made visible in ways more verbal descriptions and formal ratings could not address.

An additional benefit of this study was that the group was able to use the same expressive media as was used in the therapy. The therapists assumed that the subjective experiences from their active participation and engagement with the children and their families would lead to collaborative metaphors they created together. These collaborative metaphors would express the more general subjective experience of change experienced by all the participants in these interventions.

The inquiry began with the group creating sand trays followed by co-created fairytales to answer the questions of what it feels like to do play/expressive therapy within a government mental health agency. This experience allowed the therapists to experience the answer to the questions "What is a child's experience?", and then "What is the therapists' experience in doing creative action in this setting?". These questions were used to introduce their experiences of the unfavourable atmosphere as the larger team was applying the government request to adopt brief and more measurable outcomes for young, traumatised children. The group then used similar actions to express the case material, including the changes each therapist presented.

The intention of this project was to investigate the problem of how to include the subjective experiences of the children, families, and themselves that developed during the creative play therapies, and how this subjective experience contributed to the change all could see. The ratings and other more typical case descriptions, such as parent or teacher reports, had also indicated significant change.

The collective review by the supervision group of their arts-based expressions indicated the subjective experience of an overall positive sense of change with the supervision group. They experienced a sense of emotional joining and the emergence of a new intimacy with the families they studied. Often the images suggested a physical transformation of some sort. These images contrasted with the way the children and their families were discussed within the MDT, where the only reference to the movement was incidental or negative. Additionally, the imagery used to describe the stories of change was creative and colourful. This was also in contrast to discussion with the MDT where positive creative or expressive references seldom occurred. In summary, the arts-based expression captured a more positive tone about the experiences of change in the arts-based interventions, while the more formal descriptions did not. One conclusion was that this development of a shared positive feeling was at the heart of the change the families experienced.

The final question the supervision group addressed was "Could the arts-based material be used within the MDT?". The group asked a small number of colleagues to join them in a session in which a case was presented to them using a sand tray followed by an improvised fairytale. While the invited group did report that the expressive images were interesting and stimulated reflection, the general response was that the use of such arts-based material would be disorienting and out of place within the more formal style of the MDT. It would likely be unacceptable and be perceived in a negative light. The group decided that any such presentation would need to be very focused on a specific case and used only with unique individual professionals who were open to more creative expression and involved with the child presented.

The supervision group concluded that the use of arts-based responses to their cases was very valuable for them to understand and support the important experiences of engaging traumatised children and their families using creative playful collaborations. Their reflection was that play advances shared positive experiences as part of the change process and that this change was important despite the discouragement from the larger system they were working in. The main conclusion taken away from this experience was that these therapists needed to accept and use traditional models while not forgetting the positive experiences that come from expressive collaborations.

In both the ongoing international project and the supervision group, the participants encountered life events with highly complex social situations that included distress, hostility, and alienation. The creative collaborations provided a process to find and then focus on inner experiences that could become a new common or shared reality through the co-created metaphors.

Conclusion

Concepts such as "professional development" and "personal growth", as well as the terms "qualities", "abilities", and "skills" could be the subject of multiple definitions and countless considerations. For the purpose of this chapter, the authors decided to give priority to selected experiences and inputs considered more relevant and useful on a practical level. The examples proposed do not claim to be exhaustive, but rather, they give the reader an opportunity to relate and develop further considerations and plans of action.

Figure 7.1 shows how to conceptualise a capacity-building process, how to start and to proceed following seven steps, and how to consider two processes in a *contiguum* logic: professional development and personal growth. The two are existing from the beginning, reinforce each other over time, and the first gives progressively more space to the second. Beyond this consideration, the trainers/leaders can insert a variety of elements, and co-construct with the professionals the learning path on the basis of the needs detected, the goals to be achieved, and the starting point of the group. Each process is unique, and Figure 7.1 must be read as a benchmark adaptable to different contexts.

In the same way, the online play space dedicated to international professionals allowed the group to move within clear and safe boundaries, expressing fears and disappointment, finding new meanings in the chaos of an unpredictable and critical situation, and nurturing hope through co-constructed metaphors. The sessions were co-created by the participants and guided by improvisation, deep feelings, and creativity. As for the supervision group, it was a precious occasion for the professionals to share frustration and dissatisfaction about an unfavourable atmosphere in the working place. The group allowed time and space for the therapists to find new answers and meanings through an art-based inquiry. The inquiry resulted in an overall positive sense of change and provided new understanding and awareness for the therapists. This empowered the therapists to engage traumatised children and their families using creative playful collaborations.

In all scenarios presented, the importance given to the person (versus professional) is crucial. We find it is useful to recall some considerations shared by Wampold (2014). After examining many studies on the effectiveness of different psychotherapy treatments, he stated: "If the differences among treatments are nonexistent or are very small, are there other factors that do have an influence on the effects of psychotherapy? The answer is yes – the therapist who is providing the psychotherapy is critically important" (op. cit.: 2). The person matters, and it is on him or her and their wholeness that the investment must be made from the outset. If continually seeking to improve is one of the qualities of the effective therapist (op. cit.: 5) or professional, then in challenging circumstances this is a *necessity*. Maslow (1962: 34) stated that "no psychological health is possible unless the essential core of the person (the individual self) is fundamentally accepted, loved and respected by others and by himself".

For the authors, these words confirm the need for professionals to work on one's own person and to be supported in this process in order to be able to assist other people. In this process, play and expressive arts have a key role: through them, the whole process becomes possible and is enhanced. The experiences described in this chapter provided a safe, respectful, and consistent framework in which play and expressive arts had a positive impact on participants (and their clients) on both professional and personal levels. Individuals found a space and time to learn, developed a sense of trust and belonging to the group, and felt supported and cared for in spite of language limitations, cultural differences, and physical distance.

References

ASCD Yearbook Committee (1962) 'Creativity and openness to experience', in A.W., Combs (ed.) *Perceiving behaving becoming. A new focus for education*, Washington, DC: Association for Supervision and Curriculum Development, 141–163.

Blanco, P.J., Muro, J.H. and Stickley, V.K. (2014) 'Understanding the concept of genuineness in play therapy: Implications for the supervision and teaching of beginning play therapists', *International Journal of Play Therapy*, 23(1), 44–54.

Brooks, R. and Goldstein, S. (2015) 'The power of mindsets: Guideposts for a resilience-based treatment approach', in D., Creenshaw, R., Brooks and S., Goldstein, *Enhancing resilience in play therapy*, New York, NY: Guilford Press, 3–29.

Gil, E. (2020) *Self care for those who care for others. A career well lived, with bouts of burnout*, webinar presented for the 26th Annual Conference of the Texas Association for Play Therapy, 24 October 2020.

Halprin, D. (1999) 'Living artfully. Movement as an integrative process', in S.K., Levine and E.G., Levine (eds.) *Foundations of expressive arts therapy theoretical and clinical perspectives*, London: Jessica Kingsley Publishers, 133–149.

Harvey, S., Donovan, J. and Lamberts Van Bueren, T. (2016) 'Considerations of change in play therapy with young children', in C., Miller (ed.) *Arts therapists in multidisciplinary settings*, London: Jessica Kingsley Publishers, 123–139.

Hervey, L. (2000) *Artistic inquiry in dance movement therapy: Creative research alternatives*, Springfield, IL: Charles C. Thomas Publishers.

Inter-Agency Standing Committee and the European Commission (2021) *INFORM Risk Index 2022*, document released 31 August 2021 by the European Commission Joint Research Centre, available: https://drmkc.jrc.ec.europa.eu/inform-index [accessed 10 January 2022].

Knill, P.J., Levine, E.G. and Levine, S.K. (2005) *Principles and practice of expressive arts therapy. Toward a therapeutic aesthetics*, London: Jessica Kingsley Publishers.

Landreth, G.L. (1995) 'Self-expressive communication', in C.E., Schaefer (ed.) *The therapeutic power of play*, Northwale, NJ: Jason Aronson, 41–63.

Levine, E.G. (2005) 'The practice of expressive arts therapy: Training, therapy and supervision', in P.J., Knill, E.G., Levine and S.K., Levine (eds.) *Principles and practice of expressive arts therapy. Toward a therapeutic aesthetics*, London: Jessica Kingsley Publishers, 171–255.

Levine, S.K. (1999) 'Poiesis and post-modernism: The search for a foundation in expressive arts therapy', in S.K., Levine and E.G., Levine (eds.) *Foundations of expressive arts therapy theoretical and clinical perspectives*, London: Jessica Kingsley Publishers, 19–36.

Maslow, A.H. (1962) 'Some basic propositions of a growth and self-actualization psychology', in A.W., Combs (ed.) *Perceiving behaving becoming. A new focus for education*, Washington, DC: Association for Supervision and Curriculum Development, 34–49.

McGilchrist, I. (2012) *The master and his emissary: The divided brain and the making of the western world*, London: Yale UP, Kindle Edition.

McNiff, S. (1998) *Arts based research*, London: Jessica Kingsley.

Mochi, C. (forthcoming 2022) *Beyond the clouds: An autoethnographic research exploring the good practice in crisis settings*, Ann Arbor, MI: Loving Healing Press.

Mochi, C. and Cassina, I. (2018) *Play therapy around the globe: International crisis work with children*, training day presented at the Northwest Center for Play Therapy Studies Summer Institute, George Fox University, Portland, 6 June 2018.

Munns, E. (2000) *Theraplay: Innovations in attachment-enhancing play therapy*, Northvale, NJ: Jason Aronson, Inc.

Overseas Security Advisory Council (2020) *Venezuela 2020 crime & safety report*, 21 July 2020, available: www.osac.gov/Country/Venezuela/Content/Detail/Report/0e6ed0e0-eb8e-44cc-ab81-1938e6c8d93f [accessed 20 December 2021].

Perry, B.D. and Szalavitz, M. (2017) *The boy who was raised as a dog: And other stories from a child psychiatrist's notebook: What traumatized children can teach us about loss, love, and healing*, New York, NY: Hachette.

Rogers, N. (1999) 'The creative connection. A holistic expressive arts process', in S.K., Levine and E.G., Levine (eds.) *Foundations of expressive arts therapy theoretical and clinical perspectives*, London: Jessica Kingsley Publishers, 113–131.

Ryan, K. and Cunningham, M. (2007) 'Helping the helpers. Play therapy with children in crisis', in N.B., Webb (ed.) *Play therapy with children in crisis: Individual, group, and family treatment*, 3rd edn., New York, NY: The Guilford Press, 443–460.

Sapolsky, R.M. (2004) *Why zebras don't get ulcers: The acclaimed guide to stress, stress-related diseases, and coping*, 3rd edn., New York, NY: Holt paperbacks, Kindle Edition.

Schaefer, C.E. and Drewes, A.A. (eds.) (2014) *The therapeutic powers of play: 20 core agents of change*, Hoboken, NJ: John Wiley and Sons.

Stagnitti, K. (2021) *Learn to play therapy. Principles, process and practical activities*, Melbourne Australia: Learn to Play, available: www.learntoplayevents.com [accessed 26 January 2021].

Wampold, B.E. (2014) *Qualities and actions of effective therapists*, American Psychological Association, Education Directorate, available: https://web.archive.org/web/20190807232845/www.apa.org/education/ce/effective-therapists.pdf [accessed 16 January 2022].

Index

Note: Page numbers in *italics* indicate a figure and page numbers in **bold** indicate a table on the corresponding page. Page numbers followed by "n" indicate a note.

agent of change 1
Andronico, M.P. 104
applications (Apps) 70, 86
arts-based inquiry 4, 138, 154
arriving in Haiti 10
asylum seekers 50–66; refugee children and 50–66; status of 54, 66n1
attuned play 31
Australasia Pacific Play Therapy Association (APPTA) 72, 76
Avalanche Metaphor 51–54
Axline, V. 69, 103

Bratton, S.C. 24, 76–77
Byers, J. 28

capacity building 15; capabilities, opportunities, and choices 19–20; as a *contiguum* professional development 140–147; of local child professionals 56; role of 2, 6; in Therapeutic Play 142
case studies 60–65, 88, 111–114, 131–134; creative dialogues 41–47; family sessions 38–41
Child-Centered Play Therapy 66n5
contiguum logic 2, 4, 9, 138–139, 140–147, 156
continuous subliminal sensing 123
continuum logic 2, 9, 100
coping 16, 98, 130; in community crisis situations 38; crisis 6–7; "lack of coping capacity" dimension of Index 8
coping with the present while building for the future (CPBF) 13–24, *14*; guide to understanding and reading 15–16; lower part of 15; upper part of 15–16

Covid-19 2, 28, 37, 41–47, 69, 71–73, 84, 88, 142, 148, 150
creative arts therapies (CAT) 1–2, 148; application 37–38; integrating play with 30–35; in playroom and outside 28–48; therapeutic powers of play and 30
Crenshaw, D.A. 28
crisis 2, 6–7; contemporary crisis work, expressive arts in 6–24; Covid-19 2; Forgotten crisis 8; humanitarian perspective on 7–9; intervention 19–22; intervention, stages of *22*; therapeutic power of play and play therapy in 20–22
crisis work 2, 6–24; expressive arts in 6–24; grounding phase in 17–19
Czsikszentmihalyi, M. 124

Diamond, M.C. 53
Drewes, A.A. 28, 30
dynamic play therapy (DPT) 29

E-health 70–72, 77
Elkind, D. 97
Expressive Arts: in contemporary crisis work 6–24; in *contiguum* professional development 139; crisis intervention through 22–24; in crisis situations 17–19; in professional development and personal growth 138–157; healing elements of 139; resources for 90; therapy 1, 23
expressive momentum 32

Family Puppet Interview (FPI) 92
Floor Games 69
flow and breaks 32–33

forgotten crisis 8
form/energy balance 33

Garbarino, J. 98
General Data Protection Regulation,
    and in Australia the Privacy Act 1988
    (Privacy Act) 83
Gil, E. 35
Goleman, D. 52
good practice 2, 6, 16–17, 108, 114
grounding phase in crisis work 17–19
Guerney, B. 104
Guerney, L. 64

Haight, W.L. 102
Hanna, T. 123
Harvey, S.A. 28, 35, 152
healing power of play 1, 23, 139
Health Insurance Portability and
    Accountability Act (HIPAA) 83
high risk country 3, 8, 98–115
hot spots 34
human-induced hazards 8
humanistic play therapy skills (HPTS) 70
humanitarian perspective on crisis 7–9
Hurt, A. 80

Index for Risk Management (INFORM) 7
Inter-Agency Standing Committee
    (IASC) 7

Jennings, S. 126
journey/obstacle course 36

Kelly, E.C. 35
Kottman, T. 29

Laevers, F. 124
Landreth, G.L. 124, 139
Learn to Play Therapy (LtP) 3, 98–115;
    in classrooms 103–104; in high-risk
    countries 98–115; what and how 103
Levine, S.K. 19, 147
local support system 3, 12, 98, 145

Malchiodi, C.A. 1, 28
Maslow, A.H. 156
Masten, A.S. 104
McNiff, S. 28–29, 35, 140
Meany-Walen, K. 29
Merleau-Ponty, M. 123
metaphor 4, 30–31, 42; arts-based,
    making 38; Avalanche Metaphor 51–54;

collaborative, making 37; creative
    collaborations to co-create 147–155;
    emotional states in 34, 47; metaphorical
    conversations 34–35, 43; Theatre 2, 6,
    13; working 35
M-health 71–72
Moustakas, C. 69
movement scale 36
Mullen, J.A. 74
My Awareness Process (MAP) 2, 9, 13,
    15, 17

natural hazards 8
nature-based play therapy 120–135
neuroception 122
neuroplasticity 21

online 2, 29, 41–47; let's play . . . 90–91;
    mode of delivery 77; multiplayer gaming
    app 91; online Sand Tray 70; platforms
    86; play-space 148, 156; software
    platform 85–87; Tele-Play 89; Tele-Play
    Therapy 91–92; therapists 148–151;
    training 83
Onyochi story 115

Perry, B.D. 52
personal growth 4; in capacity-building
    process 141; *contiguum* professional
    development 139–147; play and
    expressive arts to 138–157; professional
    development and 140, 156
Piaget, J. 123, 134
play 106; across cultures 101–103;
    attunement within 31; breaks 32;
    in creative adaption and problem
    finding/solving 28; creating spaces
    to 53; developing together, with
    children 110–111; developing
    together, with teachers 107–109;
    digital game 91; embodied 126; to
    enhance professional development
    and personal growth 138–157;
    goal-oriented play-based activities
    21; integrating with the creative arts
    modalities 30–35; need for 98–101;
    for optimal learning environment 3;
    powers of, applying 105; pre-packaged
    plan of 18; projective 126; time,
    recovering lost 3, 50–66; role-play 126;
    story 112–114; therapeutic powers of
    1–3, 6–24, 30, 69–93; as a universal
    language 18, 20

playroom 130, 133, 144–145; creative arts modalities in, integrating 28–48; in-person 2; traditional 89

play therapists 1, 3–4, **78–79**, 80–81, 83, 85, 89, 93; nature-based therapeutic nurture group 126–130; Tele-Health sessions 76; in Tele-Play Therapy 69

play therapy 23, 61, 64; applying, in crisis 20; child-centred (CCPT) 50; dynamic (DPT) 29; expressive arts and 17; nature-based, interventions in digital age 120–135; non-directive 38; scaffolded telecommunications for 77–80; within the service 58–59; telecommunications for 3, 73–77; telecommunications in, contraindications for 80–81; telecommunications in, guidelines for 80; *see also* Learn to Play Therapy (LtP); Tele-Play Therapy

Porges, S.W. 122, 133

Porges' polyvagal theory 122

pretend play 63, 126, 144; abilities of children 99–100; across cultures 101–103; child's ability to, in classrooms 103; Learn to Play Therapy approach improving 108–109, 111; practice 105; *Pretend Play Enjoyment Developmental Checklist* 100; self-initiated 115; social 103; toys use in 112

Pretend Play Enjoyment Developmental Checklist (PPE-DC) 88

process of migration 51–54

process-oriented approach 2, 6–24

professional development 4, 71–72; in a capacity-building process 141; *contiguum* of 139, 140–147, 156; play and expressive arts to enhance 138

project 112–115; background 97–98; considerations and limits of 65; Developing Play Together 96, 98–99, 107–109; during Covid-19 41–47; guidelines 104–106; in India 138–157; recovering lost play time 54–60; SOS Distant Adoption Project 111; specifics 107–109; structure overview 105–107

recovering lost play time chart (RLPT chart) 53, 61, **61**

refugee children, psychosocial wellbeing of 50–66, 66n1

remote intervention 69–93; in creative arts modalities 28–48; using therapeutic powers of play 69–93

resilience 7–8, 42, 123; abilities vital for 123; baby's 125; children's, goal of improving 147; community's 8, 42; play therapy to improve 146

rituals 34

Russ, S.W. 28–29

Schaefer, C.E. 30

Schore, A.N. 125

Simard, S. 120

slow-motion races 33

software 85–87

Stern, D.N. 125, 128

Stone, J. 77

storytelling 2, 28, 33–34; children and their families engaging in 153–154; dramatic 29; importance of 35, 37

stress 6, 18–19, 43, 144, 147; in children 51–52, 66, 98, 146; chronic 97; human autonomic nervous system during 122; post-traumatic stress disorder 52, 153; relational-building competence reducing 105; self-regulation experiences to cope 106; "stress overload" situation 7

summary fairy tale 46–47

supervision 56, 83, 109, 143–145; clinical 71, 77; in CPBF approach 19; Creative Arts/Play Therapy supervision group 148; counter answer development for complexity through 152; in digital game play 91; in field work 11; in immersive VR and play therapy 87; importance of 57; individual and group 145; individual 106; play and expressive arts in 139, 153–155

supervivors 19–20

teachers 17; in creating learning environment 105; "developing play together" with 107–109; didactic teaching approach 99; enhancing capacities of 104–105; learn to play in classrooms 103–104; in practising self-regulation 106; in training 57

technological equity 84–85

Tele-Filial Therapy 73, 77, **78–79**, 89, 92

Tele-Health 70–71, 73, 76, **78–79**, 83–84, 91–92

Tele-Play 73–76, 89–90

Tele-Play Therapy 3, 69–93; Apps 86; client 81–82; consent and privacy 84; data protection compliance 83–84; disability or health conditions

85; environments preparation 81; ethico-legal considerations 83–84; financial transactions 87; geographical location 84; guiding principles 80–81; historical evolution 70–73; insurance 83; interconnected virtual settings 82; license and/or registration 83; online software platforms 86; outcomes of 92; practitioner 81; professional practice, scope of 83; resources for 90; scaffolded telecommunications for 77–80; socioeconomic factors 84–85; software considerations 85–87; technological equity 84–85; telecommunications for 73–77, 80, 82–87; Tele-Filial Therapy 77; Tele-Health 76; virtual reality (VR) 86–87

Theatre Metaphor 2, 6, 13

Therapeutic Play: capacity building in 142

therapeutic powers of play (TPoP) 55–56, 70, 71, 93, 126, 131; application of 138, 142, 146; creative arts therapies and

30; to overcome difficulties 59; remote interventions using 69–93

trauma 16, 122, 134, 147; critical situations causing 21; expressed through symbolism and metaphor 35; in families 152–156; impact of 126; intergenerational 17–18; interventions 11–12; play and the creative arts to address 28, 37, 135; social 37

United Nations Development Programme (UNDP) 19

Virtual Reality (VR) 85–87

Virtual Sandtray App (VSA) 70, 86

Vygotsky, L. 103

Wampold, B.E. 156

Webb, N.B. 7

Wells, H.G. 69

Wilson, E. 123

Winnicott, D.W. 125

For Product Safety Concerns and Information please contact our EU
representative GPSR@taylorandfrancis.com
Taylor & Francis Verlag GmbH, Kaufingerstraße 24, 80331 München, Germany

www.ingramcontent.com/pod-product-compliance
Lightning Source LLC
Chambersburg PA
CBHW060311220326
41598CB00027B/4298